Snippets in Surgery

VOLUME 2

AF778949

JP

Snippets in Surgery

VOLUME 2

Srinivasan Ravi MS FRCS(Ed) FRCS(Eng)
Former Consultant Surgeon
Blackpool Teaching Hospitals NHS Foundation Trust (BTHFT)
Lancashire, UK
Professor of Surgical Practice
KS Hegde Medical Academy
NITTE (Deemed to be University)
Mangaluru, Karnataka, India

JP medical publishers
London • New Delhi

© 2026 JP Medical Ltd.

Published by JP Medical Ltd,
83 Victoria Street, London,
SW1H 0HW, UK
Tel: +44 (0)20 3170 8910
Email: info@jpmedpub.com
Web: www.jpmedpub.com

EU GPSR Authorised Representative
Logos Europe, 9 rue Nicolas Poussin
17000, La Rochelle, France
Phone: +33 (0) 6 67 93 73 78
E-mail: Contact@logoseurope.eu

The rights of Srinivasan Ravi to be identified as the author of this work has been asserted by them in accordance with the Copyright, Designs and Patents Act 1988.

All rights reserved. No part of this publication may be reproduced, stored or transmitted in any form or by any means, electronic, mechanical, photocopying, recording or otherwise, except as permitted by the UK Copyright, Designs and Patents Act 1988, without the prior permission in writing of the publishers. Permissions may be sought directly from JP Medical Ltd at the address printed above.

All brand names and product names used in this book are trade names, service marks, trademarks or registered trademarks of their respective owners. The publisher is not associated with any product or vendor mentioned in this book.

Medical knowledge and practice change constantly. This book is designed to provide accurate, authoritative information about the subject matter in question. However readers are advised to check the most current information available on procedures included and check information from the manufacturer of each product to be administered, to verify the recommended dose, formula, method and duration of administration, adverse effects and contraindications. It is the responsibility of the practitioner to take all appropriate safety precautions. Neither the publisher nor the authors assume any liability for any injury and/or damage to persons or property arising from or related to use of material in this book.

This book is sold on the understanding that the publisher is not engaged in providing professional medical services. If such advice or services are required, the services of a competent medical professional should be sought.

ISBN: 978-1-78779-199-2

British Library Cataloguing in Publication Data
A catalogue record for this book is available from the British Library

Library of Congress Cataloging in Publication Data
A catalog record for this book is available from the Library of Congress

Project Manager: Bhavana Sharma

Editorial Assistant: Keshav Kumar Baghel

Cover Design: Seema Dogra

Typeset, printed and bound in India.

Preface

This book follows on from Snippets in Surgery (Volume 1). I have tried to maintain a similar style to that of the first volume. It is, however, pitched at a different level and addresses the needs of the trainees who are dedicated to surgery. As surgery progresses there is a need to keep up-to-date with new research publications that may make an impact on one's practice. This requires the ability to read and review ongoing publications before making a judgement on the effect of new treatments. I have, therefore, begun this edition with the basics of the scientific method with a stress on evidence-based medicine. Anecdotal evidence may vanish into thin air when confronted by evidence! The chapter on scientific methods is followed by a chapter on oncology that underpins the basics and proceeds to further chapters on cancers involving various organs. There are chapters on nutrition, metabolic response to trauma, general plastic and paediatric surgery, all of which I believe should be part of any Surgeon's Armamentarium even if she/he does not specialise in it. General plastic and paediatric surgery as well as endocrine surgery are carried out by general surgeons in many parts of the world where specialisation of the western type has not yet been introduced. When I was a trainee in India, I was exposed to all these as well as to facio-maxillary surgery and urology. This is no longer the case and delivery of specialist care has made an increasingly beneficial impact. Patients and friends are, however, likely to confront you with questions about aspects of surgery that does not pertain to your speciality and, therefore, some knowledge of basics, to me at least, seems essential for an erudite practitioner. Finally, I have discussed a few cases based on my personal experience with emphasis on the learning points. I have ended the book with multiple choice questions (MCQs) and answers followed by reflections on the progress in surgery in the last half a century.

All figures and sketches have been created by me using the Procreate application on my iPad. Through these illustrations, I have aimed to convey key concepts, operating under the principle that clarity in expression reflects clarity of understanding. Historically, I have required junior trainees to draw a diagram of the gallbladder and the common bile duct at the outset of their training. This exercise provided valuable insight into their baseline knowledge, regardless of whether they expressed interest in pursuing a career in surgery.

This book is not intended to be a treatise but can be used for rapid review and as a companion to textbooks on surgery. I understand the responsibility a single author book bestows on the author. I have been fortunate to have many colleagues who were keen to review and scrutinise many of the chapters. They are all specialists in their field. This increases the credibility of the book. The text material has been wholly the work of a single author but with many of the recommendations and suggestions implemented almost in full but within the format of a standardised text. In future editions, I intend to edit the chapters that will be written by various specialists.

This book will assist not only in the rapid and easy acquisition of key information but also reiterate and refresh knowledge. I hope you to enjoy it as much as I have in writing it.

Knowledge and skills are flip sides of the same coin and together they assist in serving the society well.

Srinivasan Ravi
November, 2025

Contributors

I wish to thank colleagues who have reviewed or contributed to various chapters of this book.

- **Chang David FRCS,** Retired Consultant Hepatobiliary Surgeon and Lead Surgeon, Department of Surgery, East Lancashire Hospitals NHS Trust (ELHT), UK. Reviewed the chapter on Hepatobiliary Cancers.
- **Debasish Debnath MS DNB FRCS Ed, FRCS(Glasg) FRCS(Eng) MD(Aberdeen) FRCS(Gen) FEBS,** Honorary Clinical Lecturer, GMC PLAB Associate Consultant, Breast and Oncoplastic Surgeon, Lancashire Teaching Hospitals NHS Foundation Trust, UK. Has reviewed the chapter on Breast Disease.
- **Ilias Marios Oikonomou MD MPhil MSt PhDc,** Specialty Doctor in General Surgery, Northwest Anglia NHS Foundation Trust, UK.
- **Jaya Ravi MSc(Physics) MSc(Computing) PGCert,** Formerly Lecturer in Computing, Blackpool Sixth Form College, UK, and my wife for reviewing the aesthetics of my sketches with critical comments.
- **Kadaba Vasudev MRCP,** Formerly Consultant Pathologist, Department of Pathology, Blackpool Victoria Hospital, UK. Reviewed the chapter on Oncology.
- **Linn Thu Ya FRCS,** Consultant Surgeon, Department of General Surgery, Blackpool Teaching Hospitals NHS Foundation Trust (BTHFT), Lancashire, UK, for his assistance with the chapters on Nutrition and Colorectal Disease.
- **Marena Gray MBBS MRCS,** Core Surgical Trainee, East of England Deanery, UK.
- **Natarajan Sivakumar MRCP,** Emeritus Consultant Dermatologist, Department of Dermatology, Newcastle Teaching Hospitals, UK. Reviewed the chapter on General Plastic Surgery.
- **Sarangan Seeralakandapalan FRCS,** Specialist Surgeon, Department of General Surgery, Blackpool Teaching Hospitals, NHS Foundation Trust (BTHFT), Lancashire, UK. Reviewed the chapter on Scientific Method to titrate level at which it is pitched.
- **Srinivasan Ravi MS FRCS(Ed) FRCS(Eng),** Former Consultant Surgeon, Blackpool Teaching Hospitals NHS Foundation Trust (BTHFT), Lancashire, UK. Professor of Surgical Practice, KS Hegde Medical Academy, NITTE (Deemed to be University), Mangaluru, Karnataka, India.
- **Stavros Gourgiotis MD PhD PGCert FRCS FACS FEBS MFSTEd,** Consultant Surgeon, Department of Upper GI Surgery, Addenbrooke's Hospital, Cambridge, UK. He and his team have shared authorship of the chapters on Upper GI and Small Bowel Cancers.
- **Susnerwala Shabbir MD FRCR,** Retired Consultant Clinical Oncologist, Rosemere Cancer Centre, Lancashire Teaching Hospital NHS Foundation Trust, UK. Reviewed the chapter on Oncology.
- **Tamilselvan Sivashanmugam FRCS,** Senior Consultant surgeon, Breast and Endocrine surgery, Associate Professor of Surgery, DSMCH, Siruvachur, Perambalur, Tamil Nadu, India. Reviewed the chapters on Endocrine Disease.
- **Vlasios Gourgiotis MSc PhD,** Student, Division of Immunology, University of Manchester, UK. Made contributions to the chapters on Upper GI Malignancies and Small Bowel Cancers.

Dedication

To the many patients whose trust and fortitude have provided invaluable learning experiences;

To my esteemed colleagues, past and present, whose professionalism and collaboration have significantly enriched my surgical journey;

To the many institutions with which I have been honoured to be affiliated, whose unwavering support and dedication to excellence profoundly influenced my professional development;

And to the students whose curiosity, commitment, and pursuit of knowledge continually inspire me to grow as an educator and professional.

I extend my sincere appreciation and dedicate this work to all of you.

Contents

Preface v
Contributors vii
Dedication ix

Chapter 1 The scientific method 1
Srinivasan Ravi

Chapter 2 Oncology 19
Srinivasan Ravi

Chapter 3 Breast disease 39
Srinivasan Ravi

Chapter 4 Upper gastrointestinal malignancies 60
Ilias Marios Oikonomou, Marena Gray, Vlasios Gourgiotis, Stavros Gourgiotis, Srinivasan Ravi

Chapter 5 Small bowel malignancies 83
Srinivasan Ravi, Ilias Marios Oikonomou, Marena Gray, Vlasios Gourgiotis, Stavros Gourgiotis

Chapter 6 Hepatobiliary malignancies 87
Srinivasan Ravi

Chapter 7 Colo-rectal disease 98
Srinivasan Ravi

Chapter 8 Thyroid disease 126
Srinivasan Ravi

Chapter 9 Parathyroid disease and calcium metabolism 137
Srinivasan Ravi

Chapter 10 Nutrition of the surgical patient 142
Srinivasan Ravi

Chapter 11 Metabolic response to trauma 152
Srinivasan Ravi

Chapter 12 General plastic surgery 158
Srinivasan Ravi

Chapter 13 General paediatric surgery 167
Srinivasan Ravi

Chapter 14 Perioperative care 171
Srinivasan Ravi

Chapter 15 Experiential case-based learning 180
Srinivasan Ravi

Chapter 16 Multiple choice questions: Test yourself 187
Srinivasan Ravi

Chapter 17 Multiple choice question: Answers 197
Srinivasan Ravi

Chapter 18 Reflections on progress in surgery – surgery then and now 204
Srinivasan Ravi

Bibliography 209

Index 213

Chapter 1

The scientific method

Srinivasan Ravi

Section 1: Introduction

In all fields of science new ideas arise. These ideas or hypotheses require *verification, validation and implementation.* Rather than using logic and authority, advances in scientific knowledge are made through gathering data and analysing the observed data and then sharing the data. This permits cross verification and confirmation of findings by others carrying out similar studies. A process by which such validation occurs is referred to as the scientific method.

The process has six steps:

1. Observation
2. Question – what one seeks to resolve
3. Hypothesis – make an assumption
4. Data – collect and collate
5. Analysis – study the results
6. Presentation and sharing of findings

If one wishes to study a new treatment option, then it is appropriate to follow the above-mentioned set of established principles that will subsequently permit sharing of information for others to replicate and verify the results. This is the modern scientific method. It was never thus. Authority held and still holds sway.

Galileo Galilei initiated the thought process, often mocking the so-called 'scientific explanations' employed by eminent philosophers of his time. He said their various explanations were *"a cloak for the correct reply which would be 'I don't know'. That reply is much more tolerable than the others as 'candid honesty' is more beautiful than deceitful duplicity".*

Roger Bacon influenced Francis Bacon, the co-founder of the scientific method and stated in his major work, opus majus (Greater work) that he considers four cardinal errors as obstacles to truth:

1. Unreliable authority
2. Custom
3. Opinion of the unskilled many
4. *Ignorance, concealed as knowledge*

Section 2: Principles of the scientific method

There is currently in scientific circles a uniform acceptance of the scientific method. The important principle in this is the formulation of a hypothesis. Without a hypothesis, any analysis is nothing more than a review of the prevailing situation. It is like looking at, for instance, the prevalence of a disease in the current population. Such information does not need a hypothesis or analysis as it is a statement of an existing fact.

Observation

Once, one makes an observation that a new treatment A, may be better than the currently available treatment B, then a question can be framed.

Question

A question that is framed will then assist in finding answers to the observation. These answers must be *measurable* and *testable.* The answers may be *numerical,* easy to measure or *behavioural* which may be more difficult. Once a question is asked, for instance, what drug is better for treating peptic ulcers, then a hypothesis can be made that can compare a H2 antagonist with a proton pump inhibitor (PPI).

A hypothesis is an untested proposition. Hypotheses are typically categorised as:

- Null hypothesis (H_0)
- Alternative hypothesis (H_a)

The null hypothesis asserts that the new intervention [e.g. a proton pump inhibitor (PPI)] does not differ from the standard treatment (such as an H2 antagonist), thereby preserving the existing condition. In this context, H_0 states: There is no difference between PPIs and H2 antagonists in managing peptic ulcers. The purpose of the study is to evaluate whether the novel intervention produces any effect, potentially beneficial, compared to current methods. Testing the null hypothesis results in two possible outcomes:

1. The null hypothesis is accepted, indicating no significant difference between treatments A and B; thus, the new therapy has no observable effect.
2. The null hypothesis is rejected, implying that treatment A is either more or less effective than treatment B.

It should be noted that terminology in this area can be ambiguous due to the prevalence of double negatives. Rejection of the null hypothesis indicates that the new approach may be superior or inferior to existing treatments.

When the null hypothesis is rejected or falsified then the treatment A and B are not the same.

The alternative hypothesis: This assumes that the new treatment is better. *This challenges the status quo.*

H_a: Treatment with PPI is better than treatment with H2 antagonists.

Alternative hypothesis makes a different assumption at the outset, and it is always opposite to that of the null hypothesis. It too requires testing against data available.

Section 3: Data and analysis

Once the null hypothesis is defined, then the information needed to refute the hypothesis is collected. Information cannot be collected from the whole population as that would be impossible. If you want to taste the salt in a cup of soup just a sip is enough to tell you if it is salty. *That is a sample.* If there is a large container full of soup, even then just a sip is still enough to tell you if it is salty! That too is a sample. The size of the sample is, therefore, independent of the size of the population to be studied but it must be sufficient to taste and be representative of the whole soup. The same applies to the value of, for instance, the blood sugar in a person. It is not necessary to bleed the entire patient to get the blood sugar level. Equally, one must ensure that the size of the sample meets the requirements of the study. One cannot sample a cup of water from the sea and conclude that there are no whales in the sea!

When observations are made from data, it is accepted that the data is uniformly spread over the whole population (be it cars, computers, plants, or people). This is called a *'normal distribution'*. The parameters when distributed 'normally' are referred to as *parametric.*

If, on the other hand, you want to look at how 'satisfied' one is with an existing treatment, the replies may be varied and unpredictable. Such types of parameters are referred to as being *nonparametric.*

Analysis

The hypothesis with the data is then subject to analysis or tests. This will depend on the type of data that is collected.

Parametric data are uniformly spread among the population and the tests used are:

- t-*test*
- z-*test* for single samples
- Paired t-*test* for paired samples
- z-*test* for independent samples

Nonparametric data are unpredictable and variable. The tests used are:

- Chi square
- Mann–Whitney
- Sign
- Binomial
- Median

Statistical studies are easier with parametric data as they fall into the *'bell curve'*. It is called the bell curve because the curve is shaped like a bell.

The bell curve follows the empirical rule, which states that 68% of the values are within one standard deviation from the mean, 95% are within two standard deviations, and 99.7% are within three standard deviations.

It is said *'there are lies, damned lies, and statistics with the bell curve'!*

The standard deviation is the deviation from the mean or median which is the summit of the curve. The standard deviation is a statistic that defines the data that is spread around the mean. Greater the data, the smaller is the deviation from the mean as all data are clustered around the mean. When the sample sizes are large the distribution curve is steep, the standard deviation as shown is small.

The Bell curve

In the early 19th century Adolph Quetelet, a Belgian mathematician, collected data on the *chest measurements* of Scottish soldiers and the *heights* of French soldiers. He introduced the concept of the average man and the body mass index (BMI). When both sets of measurements were plotted, they tended to cluster in a symmetrical shape around a mean in a graph that yielded a bell curve.

It is also called The *Gaussian curve* (**Figure 1**), after Gauss who did a lot of work on probability.

Most soldiers were in a height range close to the average. He assumed nature created human attributes around an optimal mean value but with a frequency of errors *(variations)* that was deviated around the mean.

This distribution is called *'the normal distribution'*. The deviation from the mean is the *'margin of error'.* The width of the symmetrical curve with the mean at the centre is the deviation (variance) from the mean, *'the standard deviation'* (**Figure 2**).

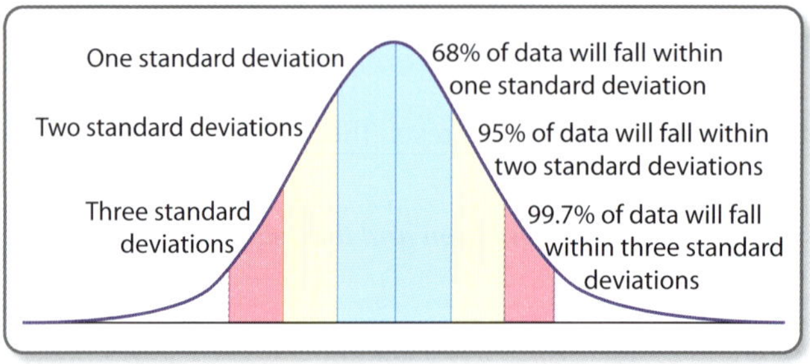

Figure 1 Gaussian distribution curve.

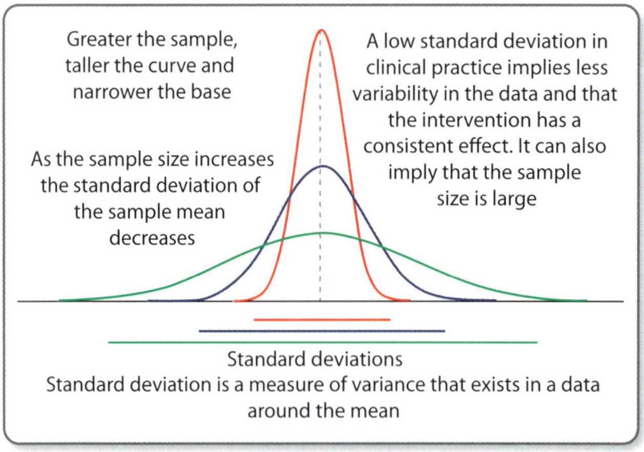

Figure 2 The standard deviation.

When the sample sizes are small, the distribution curve is wide and relatively flat. The more variable the data the larger is the standard deviation (**Figure 2**).

As the sample size increases the the standard deviation around the mean becomes narrower. As the sample size decreases the deviation is wide around the mean. It stands to reason that a low standard deviation means the sample is large. For example, with a sample size of 10, 100 and 1,000, the sample size of 10 will have a curve that will almost be flat with a wide spread around the mean. At 100 and then 1,000 the shape begins to change, and the graph increasingly becomes 'pinched' drawing the standard deviations closer at the base; this makes the *base line* between two standard deviations or three standard deviations shorter with increasing samples. *This base line represents the confidence interval.*

The 'Larger' the sample size, steeper the bell curve

The 'Steeper' the curve, narrower the base line between standard deviations

The length of the base line thus defines the strength of the data

The base line between two standard deviations is the confidence interval

The shorter the confidence interval, the larger the sample and thus the stronger the data.

Section 4: Interpretation

The impact from observations can be for the better or for the worse. Whatever the impact from observations, *we need to exclude the chance of imperfections in formulation, observation, and experiment.*

The probability that the impact of observations is not due to chance must be proven.

Significance and *p*-value

Significance is the term commonly used in statistical analysis to mean that the observed result is unlikely to be due to chance (probability). From a clinical perspective, it is of two types.

1. *Statistically significant:* The observed effect is unlikely to be due to random chance.
2. *Clinically significant:* The observed effect has an impact in practice.

For example, a cholesterol lowering drug decreases low-density lipoprotein (LDL) cholesterol by 2 mg/dL compared to a placebo. This is shown to be statistically significant at $p < 0.001$. This small result, however, is unlikely to be meaningful in practice.

p-value and probability

Imagine that we toss a coin and it falls tails. Then we toss it again and again five times. It falls tails all the time. Well, it can certainly happen twice and even thrice but four times in a row. And then we toss it a fifth time, and it falls tails yet again, we develop a strong suspicion that there is something wrong with the coin (*Gauvreau K* and *Pagano M).*

Probability

It is the study of randomness or chance in the sample of all the data that is made available. It ensures that the sample is representative of the whole data and not an error in sampling. It puts a numerical value to the sample. Normally, it is accepted that if the probability of error is <5% it is reasonable to conclude that the result was not due to chance.

Theoretically, if we toss a coin a 100 times, it is quite possible that we could get runs of five a few times. But, we did the trial just once and not a 100 times. On that first occasion, we had a run of the same face five times in a row. Something rare occurred the very first time we did it indicating that for that coin at least it may not have been a rare occurrence. In other words, the finding is significant. Therefore, we reject the null hypothesis that the coin is unbiased and accept an alternate hypothesis—that the coin is biased. [The *P*-value and Statistical Significance: Misunderstandings, Explanations, Challenges, and Alternatives (*Chittaranjan Andrade*)].

Simple mathematics tells us that the probability that a tossed coin will display the same face (heads or tails) five times in a row is 0.5 × 0.5 × 0.5 × 0.5; is, 0.0625. This *P* value, 0.0625, is rather close to the value 0.05 that is by general convention set as the cut-off for 'statistical significance' (rather than Chance).

—*Gauvreau K*

Significance only means that the result rejects the null hypothesis.

The *p*-value is always a number between 0 and 1 and interpreted in the following way:

- *A small p-value (typically ≤0.05)* indicates evidence against the null hypothesis, meaning that the treatment is better than current options. The lower the *p*-value the more significant the result in rejecting the null hypothesis.
- *A large p-value (>0.05)* indicates weak evidence against the null hypothesis, meaning that the treatment was no more effective than current treatments.

p-value is fixed before the test at a level called the significant level referred to as the Greek letter alpha (α).

If *p*-value: $p <$ or = to α we reject H_0 or the null hypothesis.

Note: To reiterate, something that is statistically significant may not be clinically significant and vice versa.

Confidence interval

It is the interval between standard deviations. It reflects the range of plausible parameters around the mean. It indicates the degree of confidence that the true mean of the parameters falls within the ranges of 68, 95, or 99.7% of the standard deviation.

If the confidence interval is 95%, it means that if the study is repeated, there is the confidence that 95% will again fall within the true mean or two standard deviations and only 5% or 1 in 20 will be outliers.

Margin of error

The value around the 'mean' that deviates from the 'mean' is the margin of error. Let us assume a sample of 100 men whose height is being measured and the mean is 175 cm. Two standard deviations will fall within a range of say 168.8 cm and 181.2 cm. This indicates that from the mean of 175 cm there is a spread on either side of the mean of 6.2 cm. The

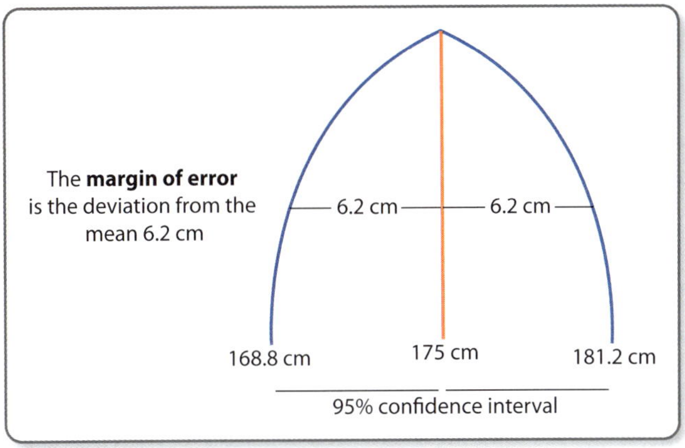

Figure 3 Margin of error.

6.2 cm is called the margin of error on either side of the two standard deviations within a 95% confidence interval (**Figure 3**).
We are confident that only 5% will be outside the range of 168.8 and 181.2 cm. If we repeat the study with 1,000 people, the two standard deviations will be narrower; the 95% confidence interval will be shorter.

Confidence interval is the equivalent of two margins of errors and plays a similar statistical role.

Confidence level

The level at which one is confident that true data has been captured is referred to as the confidence *level*. The confidence level increases with increasing margin of error.

If we were to consider three standard deviations, the confidence interval will be 99.7% indicating that only 0.3% will fall outside the confidence interval. When precision is required, *confidence level* should be low because there is requirement to be very close to the truth.

When the margin of error is high, the confidence that the data captures all probabilities is also high. Suppose one is asked to guess the number of pound coins in a bag, the confidence with which one can guess the exact number of pound coins in the bag is low when there is a requirement to be very precise and exact; however, if you are asked to guess the number of coins in the bag with an error of 5, 10, or 20 then the confidence level is highest at 20 and lowest at 0 but, the margin of error increases indicating direct proportionality between the confidence level and margin of error.

Principal steps of the scientific method

1. Ask a question and formulate a hypothesis.
2. Design a study to test the hypothesis.
3. Collect the samples for the study.
4. Set the *p* value.
5. Draw 'Conclusions' based on *p* value.
6. Null hypothesis is thus either rejected or accepted.
7. Report findings.
8. Verify by conducting similar studies.

9. A small p value negates the null hypothesis allowing us to conclude that the new treatment is better.
10. Smaller the p value, more significant the result.

Section 5: Types of studies and systematic review

Observational studies

1. *Case control:* This type of study compares a group of people with a particular condition with a group that does not. For example, smokers and nonsmokers, to try and identify a cause. For example, study of all patients with lung cancer over time to find out commonality. R Doll found that a large proportion were smokers.
2. *Case study:* A single case studied over time.
3. *Cross-sectional study:* A population study at a point in time.
4. *Longitudinal study:* Study over a period of time.
5. *Retrospective cohort study:* Uses existing data to study relationships that existed between exposures and outcomes, causes, effects, and trends in the past.
6. *Prospective cohort study:* Studies a group of people over a period of time forwards from the present.

Systematic review

Systematic review is similar to a thorough investigation, like a detective trying to get answers to a problem or a research question.

According to PRISMA Systematic reviews serve many critical roles. They can provide:

- Syntheses of the state of knowledge in a field, from which future research priorities can be identified.
- They can address questions that otherwise could not be answered by individual studies.
- They can identify problems in primary research that should be rectified in future studies.
- They can generate or evaluate theories about how or why phenomena occur.

Systematic reviews, therefore, generate various types of knowledge for different users of reviews such as patients, healthcare providers, researchers, and policy makers.

As with all reviews, it begins with a *question.* Does eating chips make you fat?

Search everywhere, in all journals, and internet for studies on this topic. Try not to miss any publication either on paper, on the internet, or in any language.

Apply a filter to get the best results based on a strict *selection* criteria, such as:

- Study design,
- Sample size,
- Quality, etc.

Extract the *data* from each study to find out how many really ate chips and how many became fat.

Combine all the data to see if chips made people fat.

Publish the result. Eating chips increases the risk of people becoming fat!

Systematic review:

- Must have well-defined inclusion criteria.

- Must summarise all available evidence.
- Must have a pre-set eligibility criterion for quality of study and methodology.

Meta-analysis

Meta-analysis can be defined as a quantitative method that mathematically combines the results from multiple studies covering the same overall topic, or the statistical pooling of the results of two or more similar studies in many languages worldwide. *[Bhandari M and Joensson A (Eds). Clin Res Surg. Verlag: Thieme; 2009.]*

1. It is the analysis of a statistical combination of the results of research studies addressing similar issues.
2. It assists in shaping guidelines that influence practice.

Systematic review gathers all the information about a particular issue. Meta-analysis crunches the numbers and provides a statistical result of multiple randomised controlled trials (RCTs) (not exclusively).

Researchers have to decide on whether to perform a systematic review or a meta-analysis depending on the question that is asked and the available evidence.

Critical appraisal

All that is published in journals and textbooks may not be true. If one needs to explore a particular topic for patient's management, the available literature could be vast.

Merriam-Webster thesaurus states that appraisal, assessment, estimation, evaluation, rating, and valuing all mean *'to judge something with respect to its worth or significance.'*

Critical appraisal can be applied to different types of studies such as:

- Systematic reviews
- Observational studies, such as cohort and case studies
- Randomised control studies

The process of critical appraisal:

- Seeks out published material
- Filters the available evidence
- Presents a condensed report that is easy to understand.

The process starts with asking the right question and seeking out published studies and validating it by scrutinising:

- Study design
- Bias
- Quality of reporting
- Statistical issues
- Outcomes

This permits one to evaluate the trustworthiness and value of a publication for implementation in one's practice for the benefit of the patient.

Summary

Critical appraisal: Can I trust this study? Was the randomisation done properly, were patients similar at the baseline, were the outcomes clinically relevant and are the results applicable to my patients.

Systematic review: What does the evidence say? Do statins reduce cardiovascular events in T2D? Search publications in pubmed, Cocharane, etc. and include only high quality RCT's, etc. Conclude, that statins do reduce cardiovascular events.

Meta analysis: How big is the treatment effect? Yes statins show a 22% relative risk reduction in cardiovascular mortality. Narrow confidence intervals indicating strong evidence.

According to Cochrane UK, critical appraisal is the highest form of knowledge in science and plays a fundamental role in evidence-based healthcare.

Preferred reporting items for systematic reviews and meta-analyses

Preferred reporting items for systematic reviews and meta-analyses (PRISMA) is a reporting guideline designed to address reporting of systematic reviews.

It is an evidence-based minimum set of items for reporting in systematic reviews and meta-analyses.

PRISMA focuses on the reporting of reviews evaluating randomised trials but can also be used as a basis for reporting systematic reviews of other types of research, particularly evaluations of interventions (Prisma.org) (**Figures 4 and 5**).

The PRISMA statement was published in 2009 and revised in 2020. It consists of a checklist and a flow diagram.

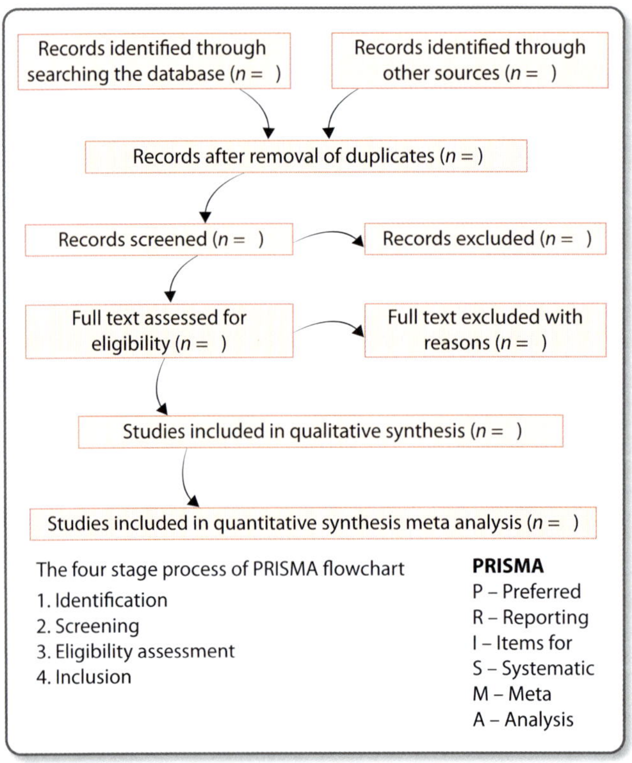

Figure 4 Preferred reporting items for systematic reviews and meta-analyses (PRISMA).

Step 1 Database search identifies 10,000 records | Additional search identifies 1,000 records

Step 2 5,000 **duplicate** records removed

Step 3 **Screening** removes another 4,500

Step 4 500 full text document assessed for **eligibility**

Step 5 400 full text documents **excluded:**
- Lack of follow-up details
- Inability to translate or retrieve
- Non-curative surgery
- Unrelated recurrences
- Insufficient numbers
- Duplicate data

100 included in quantitative synthesis (meta-analysis)

Meta anaysis as a 'study of studies' when done well is a pre-eminent basis for evidence-based delivery of care

Figure 5 An example of a preferred reporting items for systematic reviews and meta-analyses (PRISMA).

Using the PRISMA checklist and guidance, publications in all languages can now be analysed and evaluated statistically and reported. The tool normally used to provide a graphic representation of a meta-analysis is called a *Forest plot.*

It is called a forest plot because the final presentation has a 'forest of lines.' It is the statistically analysed final report of multiple studies asking similar questions and providing results.

Interestingly a forest plot is the logo of the Cochrane Trust, a UK charity committed to meta-analysis of RCTs.

The results of the individual studies in the systematic review may be varied and will have different confounders. The selection of reports for studies can be done with the aid of PRISMA chart. The basic question is asked and reports from around the world are studied. Reports that do not fit the criteria are excluded. Reports from various languages, not only in the English language, are included. Finally, a filtered group of studies are analysed statistically. The pooled result is then reported in a uniform manner using the 'Forest plot.' Effectively, it is a final representation of a study of studies.

Section 6: Presentation of results

The Forest plot (Figure 6)

In the 'Forest plot,' the names of the studies in the systematic review are represented in chronological order on the left of the graph.

To the right of the names of authors in chronological order there is representation of the study in terms of the investigated group and control group. This is presented as 'n/N.'

- n – number with events
- N – the total number

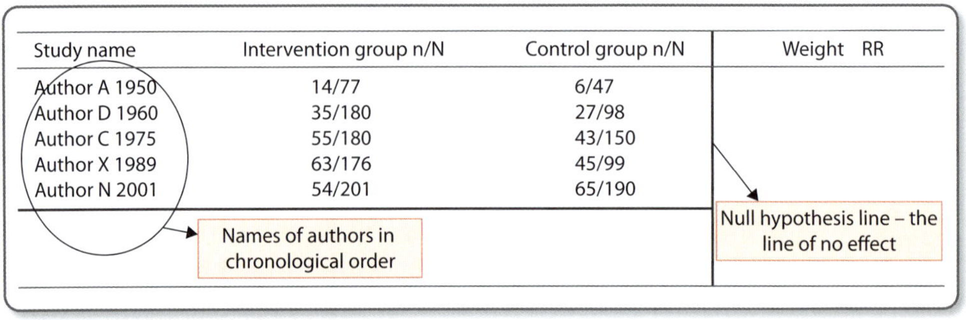

Figure 6 The 'Forest plot': *presentation of results.*

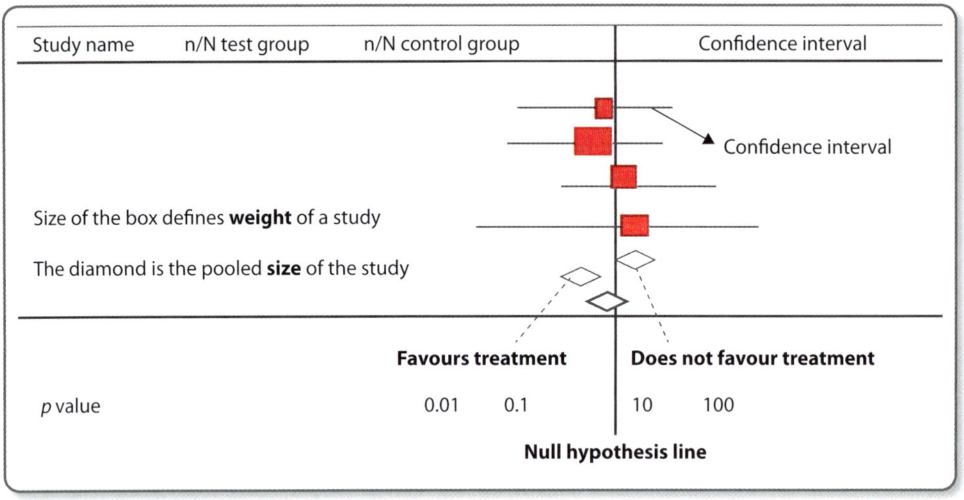

Figure 7 Possible locations of the diamond.

A vertical line represents the 'LINE OF NO EFFECT'.

Weight of each study may also be included in the 'Forest Plot'. At a glance, this will provide the effect that the study had on the pooled result that is represented as a '*diamond*'.

The sixth column showing the relative risk can be shown as numerical values. This is also expressed as a box in the 4th column and is expressed in numbers.

The picture shows three possible locations of the diamond (**Figure 7**). The next column visually displays the study results. The boxes show the effect estimates from the single studies, while the diamond shows the pooled result.

The horizontal lines through the boxes illustrate the length of the confidence interval. As we have seen, the longer the lines the wider the confidential interval, and less reliable the study results. The larger the study the shorter the horizontal line representing the confidence interval.

The most valuable is the diamond.

If a horizontal line is drawn across the diamond, it represents the collated confidence interval. If a line is drawn across the vertical summits of the diamond that line represents point estimate of the averaged studies.

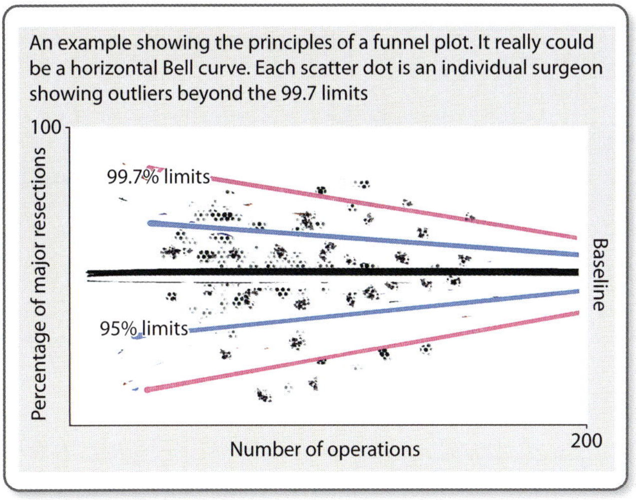

Figure 8 The 'Funnel plot'.

The vertical line of no effect or the null line is the position at which there is no clear difference between the intervention group and the control group.

If the diamond touches or crosses the null line, then the study has not disproved the null hypothesis.

The 'Forest plot' is thus a visual representation that shows the effect of the meta-analysis at a glance.

Funnel plot

The other type of representation is by a scatter plot referred to as the 'Funnel plot' because of the way it is represented. The representation is visual with each study being represented as a dot. The 'X' axis shows the mean result and the 'Y' the size of the sample. Outliers can be picked up on the visual representation at a glance (**Figure 8**).

The Kaplan–Meier curve

In 1958, Edward L. Kaplan and Paul Meier collaborated to publish a seminal paper on how to deal with incomplete observations. The Kaplan–Meier curves are used in medical literature to display cancer survival times in an easy to understand and compare graph. Time is plotted on the 'X' axis and time to event be it death or other events is plotted on the 'Y' axis. Comparisons can be made based on the shapes of the curves. If the curves are parallel, then the results indicate similar survival than if they diverge (**Figure 9**).

Levels of medical evidence

Ia: Meta-analysis of randomised control trials
Ib: Randomised control trial
IIa: Well-designed controlled study without randomisation
IIb: Well-designed quasi-experimental study
III: Well-designed case studies, comparative and correlative studies
IV: *Expert committee reports, opinions of experts and respected authorities*

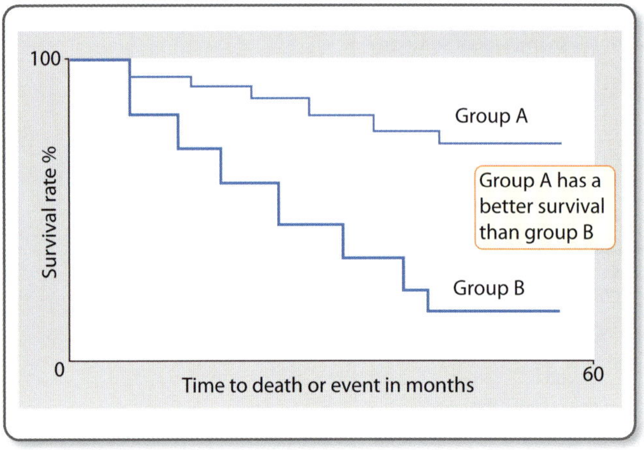

Figure 9 The Kaplan–Meier curve.

Grading of recommendations:

1. Grade A: Needs at least one good quality RCT
2. Grade B: Needs clinical studies without randomisation
3. Grade C: Evidence from category 4

Note that the least valued are opinions of individual experts without proper scientific backing!

Section 7: Key information regarding benefits and harms

Benefits and harms are difficult to quantify for any single person. Statistical guidance may assist the clinicians in the decision-making process.

A system of working out the benefit/harm for any individual patient is based on the number of patients one needs to treat for one patient to benefit.

For instance, the numbers needed to be treated (NNT) figure for one person to benefit from thrombo-embolic deterrent (TED) stockings and prevent deep vein thrombosis (DVT) is 7. This means that one DVT can be prevented by application of the TED stockings. Six persons will have used it for no benefit.

This again depends on the starting point or base-line risk of a person getting the DVT. As the base-line risk increases, the number needed to be treated for one benefit decreases.

Another example is aspirin and prevention of myocardial infarction. If the base-line event risk such as myocardial event is predicted to be low at 0.5% per year, then the number of patients needing treatment for one person to benefit is 133 (Bandolier). As the base-line risk increases to 1.5% cardiac event per year, the NNT for one person to benefit is 44. For this latter group, the numbers needed to cause harm such as a major bleed is 53.

Numbers needed for benefit and harm are critical judgements that should ideally be considered for each patient and each situation. The base-line risk must be assessed as the benefits of treatment increase with increasing risk.

Risk reduction is a way of assessing benefits of one type of treatment allowing for comparison between treatments for the same prevalence of base line risk.

Example:

Absolute risk	AR
Absolute risk reduction	ARR
Relative risk	RR
Relative risk reduction	RRR
Control event rate	CER
Experiment event rate	EER
Numbers needed to treat	NNT
Numbers needed to harm	NNH

In this example (**Table 1**), 50 people must be treated for 1 person to benefit from it. 49 people will have no benefit but can come to harm from the side effects.

Relative risk reduction though often quoted in studies is not as reliable as *absolute risk reduction*. The numbers quoted for relative risk reductions most often seem to be large. RRR appears impressive as it magnifies improvement but not clinical impact. RRR states proportional effectivity of a treatment. It is only ARR and NNT that state the clinical effectiveness. It is also dependent on the 'starting point' or baseline risk. It can be calculated the easy way by subtracting the relative risk from 1. Depending on what the study is about, a risk of <1 will signify a greater impact of the treatment.

As the numbers appear larger than ARR one can become convinced of the benefits of drug A over B. In these situations, it is best to scrutinise the absolute risk reduction and use the reciprocal to assess the NNT. Over time, if this becomes a habit, there will be a clearer understanding of this type of information.

Table 1 50 persons must be treated for 1 to benefit in this example.

Experimental group size	100
Control group size	100
Events in experimental group (EER)	1
Events in control group (CER)	3
AR in experimental group	1
AR in control group	3
Calculations	
ARR = CER – EER	2
RR = EER/CER	1/3 = 0.33 = 33%
RRR = CER – EER/CER	(3 – 1)/3 = 2/3 = 0.67 = 67%
RRR = 1 – RR	1 – 0.33 = 0.67 = 67%
NNT = 1/ARR	1/2, i.e. 50 patients

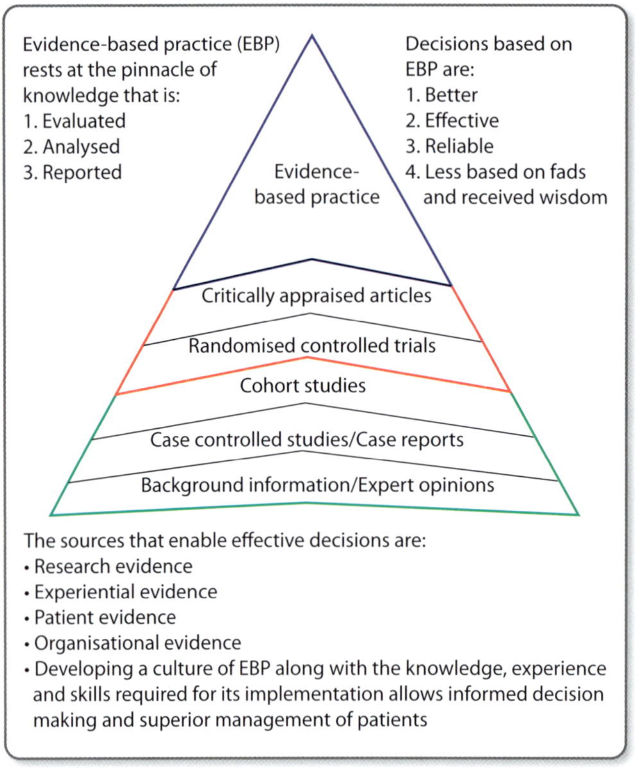

Figure 10 Evidence-based practice.

Section 8: Evidence-based practice (Figure 10)

Evidence-based practice (**Figure 10**) when followed will lead to management of all patients in such a way as to reduce the risks and increase the benefits of care. Such a system is based on a number of key factors:

1. *Systematic review of research:* Studies of high-quality reliable evidence identifies best practice and helps to ensure that decisions are based on the best available data.
2. *Critical appraisal:* Evaluating the quality and relevance of research studies ensures that they are credible and applicable to a specific context.
3. *Clinical guidelines:* The developing and following of clinical guidelines based on evidence-based recommendations for practice assists in delivery of standardised care that reduces variability.
4. *Risk-benefit analysis:* Weighing the potential benefits of an intervention against the potential risks helps in making informed decisions that prioritise patient's safety.
5. *Patient's involvement:* Engaging patients in decision-making is essential for understanding their preferences and concerns, helping to tailor interventions and minimise harm.
6. *Ongoing monitoring and evaluation:* Continuously evaluating the results of interventions and making necessary adjustments is essential to ensure patient's safety and treatment efficacy.

7. *Interdisciplinary collaboration:* This approach involves accommodating ideas from different teams of healthcare professionals, bringing diverse perspectives and expertise to decision-making, which can help to identify and mitigate potential risks.

These strategies help to create a systematic and thoughtful approach to delivering care, ensuring that decisions are not only effective but also prioritise patient's safety and well-being.

Section 9: Reading a paper

"We are drowning in information but starved for knowledge."

—John Naisbitt

Based on the discussions hitherto, reading, analysing and assessing any publication should be a matter of stepwise progression to the ultimate question, *will the material presented change my practice?*

To do this it is good to follow a concise *'Why, How and What guide':*

Why was the study done? Skim read the paper by reading the title, authorship, abstract and conclusion to grasp the central idea.

How has it been done? Understand the structure.

IMRaD:
- Introduction
- Methods
- Results
- Discussion

Herman Ebbinghaus wrote a paper on memory in 1885. In this he drafted the first standardised report. He arranged his paper into the IMRaD format. This format was so impressive that it has now become accepted as the standard for all publications.

Focus on key aspects of methods, results and conclusion

Critically analyse the methodology.
- Are the data collection methods explained in sufficient detail?
- Which methods were employed to analyse the data?
- What quality control measures were implemented?
- Was the appropriate technique utilised?

What is the conclusion?
- Do the results support the conclusion?
- Stick to facts and avoid opinions.
- Identify biases.
- Note limitations.
- Are the results transferable to other clinical settings?

Discussion

This section of any publication is pivotal to the article as it addresses the research questions and presents the significance of the analysis and interpretation of the data. Typically, the results of the study are compared with those from other studies, emphasising the differences or similarities. Generally, no new data is introduced in this section; instead, it focusses on reiterating key points from previous sections.

References/Bibliography

Scan through it and ensure that there is a complete listing of the sources from which the information was obtained.

The ability to read a paper well enables clinicans to practice evidence based medicine by critically appraising validity and relevance, leading to safer patient care and better clinical decisions.

Chapter 2

Oncology

Srinivasan Ravi

Section 1: The cell cycle

"Advances are made by answering questions; discoveries are made by questioning answers"

—*(Bernhard Haisch 1975)*

The term 'cancer' comes from the Greek word 'Karkinos', meaning crab. Hippocrates first referred to it, comparing a cancerous growth to a crab's hard shell and tentacles.

'It is a disease caused by the uncontrolled growth of a single cell. This growth is unleashed by mutations - changes in DNA that specifically affect genes that incite unlimited cell growth. In a normal cell, powerful genetic circuits regulate cell division and cell death. In a cancer cell, these circuits have been broken, unleashing a cell that cannot stop growing. That this seemingly simple mechanism - cell growth without barriers - can lie at the heart of this grotesque and multifaceted illness is a testament to the unfathomable power of cell growth.' So, writes, Mukherjee, Siddhartha in his superb book, The Emperor of All Maladies.

Cell division is a universal principle that enables life. Without it living beings cannot grow or recover from injury. It forms the substratum on which all repair and remodelling occurs after inflammation. It is a surrogate marker of life. Replication is obviously prone to errors but considering the billions of cells in our body a replication error occurs only once in 10,000 replications. These are corrected making the true value more like one error in 20,000 replications or more. Even so, given that there are billions of cells, this can lead to problems. The cell that recognises its error commits 'hara-kiri' or suicide. A process called 'apoptosis.' This process is facilitated by 'P53.' P53 is a suppressor gene present in chromosome 17 and is referred to as the guardian of the genome. Sadly, it is mutated in most cancers.

Cell division is not a rapid process in human beings and unlike bacteria which are 'pregnant even as they are born', cell division is a meticulous, laborious, and pre-programmed process that takes time. For most cancer cells it takes about 40–220 days.

All cells arise from cells and the time that it takes for one cell to become two and two to become four is called the *doubling time*. Once the cells have replicated, not all of them continue to replicate and grow. Some cells stop growing and go into a dormant phase.

Rudolph Virchow is acknowledged as the father of 'modern pathology'. He made the link between cell growth and cancer.

Most famously, Virchow is credited with *the third principle of cell theory.* Cells were first described by Hooke, in 1665, when he likened them to 'cella' or small room, much like the rooms inhabited by monks of the time. Internal components could not be seen and so there was no presumption that they were alive! The cell theory is attributed to Schleiden and Schwann in 1839 and Virchow contributed to it.

The theory put forward may seem simple today but in the 1800s, it was still a revolutionary concept. Antonie van Leeuwenhoek had written to Hooke, who was the President of the Royal Society, stating that with his improvement of the magnification of the microscope, he had seen things far surpassing that which he had seen before. The fact that 'animalcules' or little animals (bacteria) were seen by Leeuwenhoek, did not automatically lead to the now established conclusions of the cell theory that:

1. All living things are composed of cells.
2. The cell is the basic unit of structure in organisms.
3. *Cells arise from pre-existing cells (Virchow)*

Omnis cellula et cellula – all cells from cells. Having established this concept, Virchow looked at malignant cells and cell growth. He noted that cells grew fatter – *hypertrophy,* or they increased in number – *hyperplasia.* Some grew without control and seemed to have a mind of their own (see **Box 1**). He called it '*neoplasia*'.

Box 1 Pathological principles.

- Hypertrophy: Increase in cell *size*
- Hyperplasia: Increase in cell *numbers*
- Metaplasia: Change of cell type
- Dysplasia: Presence of abnormal shape, size, or order of cells
- Neoplasia: *Abnormal new* growth of cells
- Anaplasia: *Loss of differentiation* to embryological state of multiplication
- Metastasis: *Migration* of cancer from one area to another.
  Meta = beyond; *Stasis* = stillness

Note: The three embryological parts of the body are:

1. Endoderm
2. Ectoderm
3. Mesoderm

- Squamous carcinoma: Arises from ectodermal squamous epithelium – such as the skin
- Adenocarcinoma: Arises from endodermal columnar epithelium
- Sarcoma: Arises from *mesodermal* structures such as muscles

The ectodermal layer is on the exterior of the embryo, the endodermal layer lines the interior, and the mesoderm is the middle layer much like the content of a sandwich. As you can see from the above, the types of epithelia are distinct for these three layers. In general, they give rise to three different types of malignancies.

The cell cycle

All cells replicate (**Figure 1**). This permits *repair and regeneration.* Cells switch from the phase of *replication* to *resting* referred to as G_0. When the cells are cycling, they can be affected by chemotherapeutic agents just as a cyclist on the road, can be hit by a truck but not normally one that is parked in a garage. The period spent in the garage is one of *dormancy.*

G_1 and G_2 are gap phases and S is the synthesis phase where DNA is synthesised.

M – Mitosis is when replication or doubling occurs with the formation of another identical cell. An amazing process with errors being corrected by *'Mismatch repair genes (MMR)'.* The DNA mismatch repair system is a highly sophisticated system that corrects biosynthetic errors that occur during replication by a process of surveillance. Where the MMR system is faulty and rectification of errors fail, apoptosis or cell death (suicide) is promoted by *P53* thus destroying the abnormal cell. This occurs normally on a regular basis in all biological systems. Where MMR is faulty, cancers may arise. This is common in colorectal cancers. If *P53* is mutated, the process of apoptosis will be defective, and the abnormal cell will then continue to flourish leading to cancer. Where a defect gives the cell an advantage such as a *gain of function* it will grow at the cost of other cells and a runaway cell is born initiating a malignant process.

P53, the guardian of the genome, facilitates apoptosis when errors in replication are noted. It is mutated in most cancers.

Mismatch repair genes can also be mutated. Their mutation is recognised by the presence of abnormalities in short sequences of nucleotide bases within the genome. Microsatellite is a short, repetitive sequence of DNA made up of the same nucleotides repeated many times in a row, such as A A A A A A. They are present in the normal DNA and are scattered throughout the genome. During replication, polymerase, can slip on these repeated sequences and extra repeats can be added or lost. Normally, *MMR* genes fix these repairs.

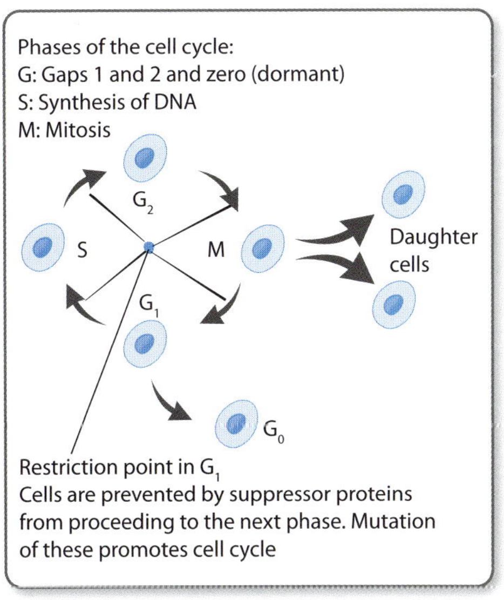

Figure 1 The cell cycle.

DNA replication during cell division is prone to error.

The rate at which incorrect nucleotides are added during DNA replication is the *spontaneous mutation rate.*

Control of DNA repair is closely tied to regulation of the cell cycle. Cells transit through a cycle involving the G_1, S, G_2, and M phases, with DNA replication occurring in the S phase and mitosis in the M phase.

During the cell cycle, checkpoint mechanisms ensure that a cell's DNA is intact before permitting DNA replication and cell division to occur. Failures in these checkpoints can lead to an accumulation of damage, which, in turn, leads to mutations.

Source: Clancy S. DNA damage and repair: mechanisms for maintaining DNA integrity. Nat Edu. 2008; 1(1):103.

If however, they themselves are mutated, then the replication error is not corrected. The length of the repeated segments changes, leading to microsatellite instability (MSI). PCR (polymerase chain reaction) test for MSI looks at the length and quantifies it as MSI-high, MSI-low or MSS (stable).

Normal cells being 'mortal' cannot multiply indefinitely. *Hayflick,* an American Scientist, in 1961, was researching into cancer cells to find out if cancer can be transmitted by contact between one cell and another.

When Hayflick grew the human cells on a plate, he saw that the cells multiplied 50–70 times and then they stopped multiplying. He repeated the experiment by growing old and young cells together and found that the old cells stopped multiplying once the 50–70 replications were reached. This came to be called the *Hayflick limit.*

On the other hand, *HELA* cells named after 'Henrietta Lacks' whose cervical cancer cells were donated to research when cultured, on a plate, continued to replicate infinitely; *they are cancer cells and are immortal.* HELA cell cultures are used for research purposes all over the world.

In 1983, a Russian scientist, *Alexi Olovnikov,* came up with the idea that the Hayflick limit was due to the gradual shortening of telomeres. *Telomeres* are the specific DNA-protein structures found at both ends of each chromosome gathering this complex structure into a tight ring like at the end of a shoelace. A small portion of telomeric DNA is lost with each cell division. When telomere length reaches a critical limit, the cell undergoes *senescence and/or apoptosis.* As telomeres shorten, they permit oncogenic transformation. Specific lifestyles may expedite telomere shortening by inducing damage to DNA in general or more specifically to telomeres and may, therefore, affect health and lifespan of an individual.

Section 2: Neoplasia – the classical theory of cancer

Neoplastic cells arise through a process of:

- Initiation: Ignition to start the car
- Promotion: Acceleration
- Progression: Drive away

It has been recognised that certain chemicals can initiate DNA abnormality. This is mostly corrected *but a single cell may retain the unrepaired DNA.* Following this, with repeated exposure to a promoter, referred to as a carcinogen, there occurs a proliferation of *clones.* This expansion of abnormal cells is called *clonal expansion*. In the progression phase, additional genetic mutations occur leading to cancer.

The two-stage model of Moolgavkar, Venzon and Knudson:

Initiation is the first step. A carcinogen damages the DNA of a cell, causing a mutation that could potentially lead to cancer development if not repaired.

Promotion is the second step. A promoting agent (not necessarily a carcinogen itself) can stimulate the mutated cell to rapidly divide and become cancerous.

This states that there are three compartments.

- Normal stem cells
- Intermediate cells that have been altered by one genetic event
- Malignant cells that have been altered by two genetic events

The size of each compartment is altered by rates of transition between:

- Cell birth
- Cell death
- Cell differentiation

Knudson's two-hit hypothesis (Figure 2)

This is different from the two-stage theory. We inherit one allele for each autosomal gene from each parent. The normal allele is referred to a 'wild type' and the abnormal allele as 'mutant'. One of the alleles can be inherited as a mutant. Retinoblastoma is caused by two mutations, one in each copy of a single tumour suppressor gene (now called *RB1*). The general population accumulates RBI mutation over the years. Knudson noted, however, that in patients with an inherited RB1 mutation (*first hit*) in one allele, tumours occurred earlier due to the acquired mutation (*second hit*). Both alleles must be mutant for cancer to occur. When both alleles are wild type, it takes longer for environmental factors to induce mutations in both alleles than it would if one allele were already inherited as a mutant.

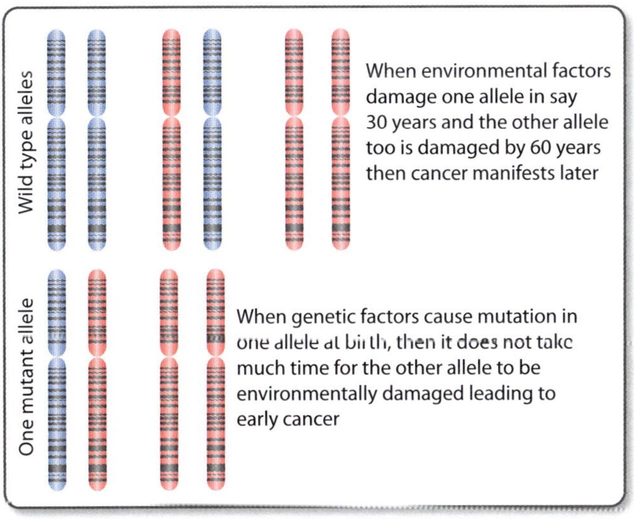

Figure 2 Two-hit hypothesis.

The *promoter* may be:

- Hormones such as oestrogen in breast cancers
- Drugs
- Infective agents
- Chemicals

The process of initiation does not lead to malignancy per se. There is a need for other factors to enable it to progress to a malignant lesion overtime.

Correlated factor such as *smoking* is associated with lung cancer, however, *correlation is not causation*. Not all patients who smoke get lung cancers but a significant proportion of them (15–20%) do. This makes it clear that while there is a strong correlation between lung cancer and smoking it is clearly not the sole factor.

Factors involved in causation of cancer

The cause of most cancers is currently unknown. There are a few cancers with known causative agents but in principle the factors involved in carcinogenesis are:

- *Agent* – known carcinogens. The most obvious is *sunlight* and radiation
- *Chemicals* and *infections* can also act as agents. Some examples are human papillomavirus (HPV) and *H. pylori* infections.
- *Hormones* – oestrogen and breast/endometrial cancer, but many remain elusive.
- *Virus* – they account for about 10% of all cancers. HPV as stated above but Epstein–Barr (EB) virus, Simian virus and Rous sarcoma virus are all linked to cancers by their ability to incorporate their genes into the host DNA.
- *Host factors* – susceptibility due to immune or genetic status. Presence of chronic inflammation, high body mass index (BMI), and diabetes
- *Environment* – many suspected factors but only few are positively proven. Asbestos exposure and mesothelioma, tobacco and lung cancer and soot in chimney sweep cancers of the scrotum as initially observed by Sir Percival Pott.

'Cancer' is now known to be a genetic disease.

In tumour development, cell nuclei undergo mutations, which can result in cytologically visible chromosome aberrations. David Hansemann (1858–1920) and Theodor Boveri (1862–1915) were major contributors to early debates on the relationship between chromosomal defects, tumourigenesis and malignancies. In 1890, Hansemann observed asymmetrical nuclear divisions in human epithelial cancers. In these abnormal, but bipolar, divisions, a fraction of the chromosomes fails to segregate properly. Boveri's central tenet was the somatic mutation theory of cancer, a tumour typically originates from a single cell that has inherited a defined, but incorrectly combined, set of chromosomes.

Tumour growth curve (Figure 3)

- Tumours grow by doubling of the cells.
- The doubling time is the time taken for one cancer cell to become two.
- Cells can be active or dormant.

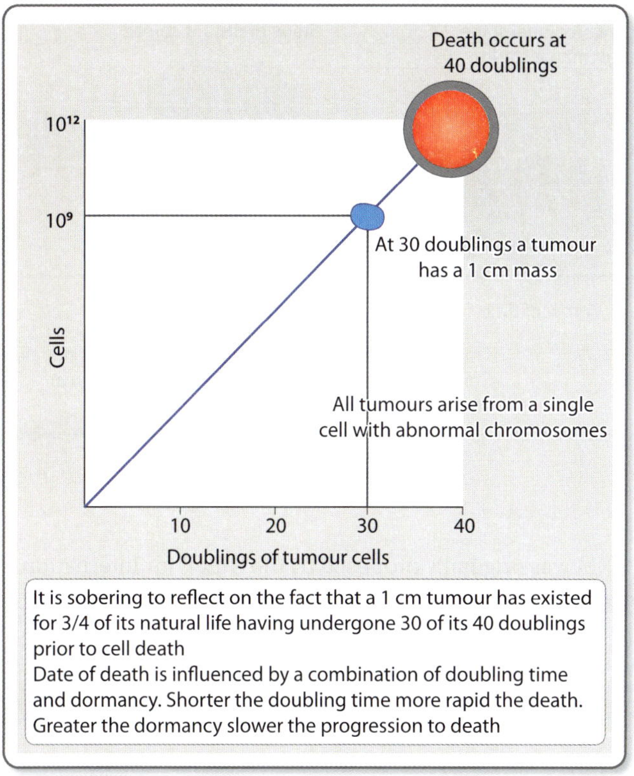

Figure 3 The tumour growth curve doubling dormancy, and death.

- Tumour growth is a balance between doubling and dormancy.
- Metastases grow faster and have a shorter doubling time.

Tumour diameter coincides with cell diameter. Assuming the earliest macroscopic lesion has a diameter of 1 mm^3, 20 doublings will be necessary to reach this size. When 10 additional mitotic divisions occur, tumour volume becomes 1 cc. After 30 doublings, then, the initial single cell tumour has become a 1 cm lesion. When the number of doublings equals 40, extensive disease is present as it equals 1 kg of tissue. Death soon follows after a few more doublings.

(Mordecai Schwartz D. Cancer. Wiley Online Library. 1961.)

The above hypothesis is purely mathematical. The rates of doubling of cancer cells are very variable and metastases grow faster. Nevertheless, while the doubling times are variable, the number of doublings needed for a tumour to become detectable shows that at the time of detection, it has been present for a considerable time.

A 1 cm tumour as can be seen has probably existed for many years before recognition.

Section 3: Tumour staging

This is a concept built on progression of rapidly uncontrollably multiplying cells from *undetectable* to *detectable* to *distant.*

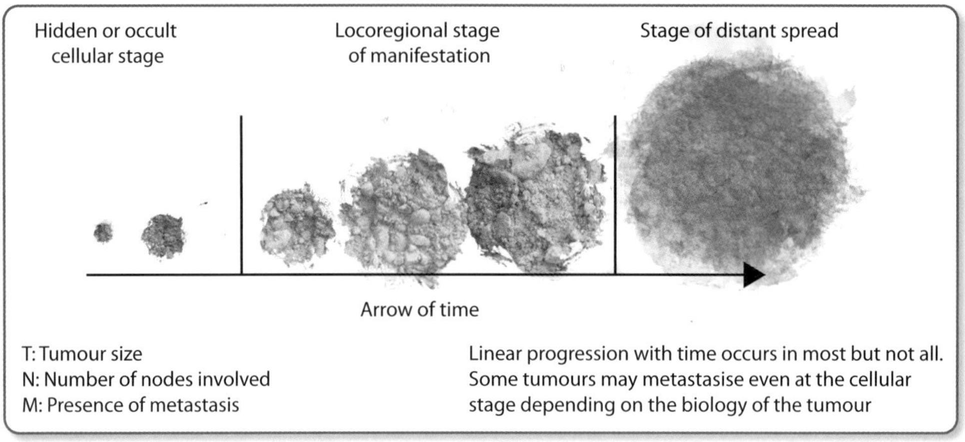

Figure 4 Tumour growth over time.

*TNM (**Figure 4**):* The staging of TNM was originally proposed by the Union for International Cancer Control (UICC) as a unified standard. The UICC works closely with the World Health Organisation (WHO).

The agreed usage of TNM across all tumour sites allows comparison of quality of care between countries and centres. It facilitates treatment of planning and prognostication.

Tumour grading

Grading a tumour is different from staging a tumour.

- The grading is about how malignant a tumour is
- The staging is how widely spread it is.

  Grading is based on cells and their change.
  Staging is based on histology and their spread.

Just as staging is categorised by the TNM staging, the cellular propensity to malignant spread can be graded by:

- *The size of the nucleus* – as the DNA unfolds during reversal to replication as opposed to specialised function, the nucleus becomes larger. The nuclear - cytoplasmic ratio moves in favour of the nucleus.
- *The number of malignant looking cells per high power field* – this is the *Broder's classification.* Broders originally proposed a four-grade system based on the percentage of undifferentiated malignant cells ranging from 25 to 100%. Broders' system is historical. Modern pathology simplified grading for practicality and most current systems use 3 grades (good/moderate/poor)

The grading is based on exfoliative cytology. Malignant cells lose their stickiness and, hence, can be retrieved mechanically by spatula – as from cervical smears or by washouts as in lungs and stomach or by needle aspiration as in breast and thyroid. On placing the cells on a slide, they can be studied for their character. This was first recognised by *George Papanicolaou* when he was studying the changes to vaginal epithelium during menstrual cycle. This led the way for 'Pap smear' and 'screening for cervical cancer'.

The roots of precision cancer therapy began at the Mayo Clinic in 1914 when surgical pathologist *Albert C.* Broders began collecting data showing that cancers of the same histologic type behaved differently. In March 1920, based upon 6 years of clinical follow-up, Broders published his first paper, utilising data from over 500 cases of squamous cell carcinoma of the lip that he had blindly divided into four histologic grades based upon degree of differentiation, showing that numerical tumour 'grading' allowed him to predict patient's prognosis.

Before this, surgeons had no scientific way to evaluate prognosis. Broders then replicated his work using other types of tumours at other body sites, as did several Mayo Fellows and pathologists at other institutions.

Cuthbert Dukes in London, England, not only replicated Broders' findings with rectal adenocarcinomas, but he also used the same data to develop the first tumour 'staging' methodology by focusing upon depth of local invasion and presence or absence of lymph node metastases. Soon, tumour grading, tumour staging, or the combination of both represented state-of-the-art prognostic techniques for scientific cancer care.

Section 4: Factors driving cancer

Genetic mutations

These can be inherited or acquired.

- *Germline mutations* occur at or before fertilisation and are thus transmitted as an inherited defect.
- *De novo mutation* as the name suggests occurs spontaneously in the sperm or ovum and there may be no history of cancer in the previous generations.
- *Somatic mutations* are more common and occur in the cell during growth.

These mutations confer a selection of advantage leading to preferential growth of the mutated cell. This results in rapid growth of a set of cells or clones – clonal evolution and selection. As these cells acquire a growth advantage by a single mutation, they soon outgrow neighbouring cells. It is possible that a second mutation can arise in this clone and the cycle is repeated leading to clonal expansion. The process of mutation and expansion progresses leading to disorganisation ultimately conferring it the ability to invade and metastasise.

Key steps in the process leading to malignancy

1. Mutation – germline/de novo/somatic
2. Clonal evolution conferring growth advantage to some cells
3. Clonal expansion is when more mutations occur within the clones leading to increased growth
4. Disorganisation
5. Invasion when malignant cells breach the basement membrane
6. Metastases where there is spread to other tissues

The mutations can be of many types:
- Point mutations
- DNA rearrangement
- DNA amplification
- DNA deletion
- Altered DNA methylation

Functional consequences of mutations:
1. Gain of function
2. Loss of function

Gain of function mutations (*accelerator*) leads to activation or acceleration and includes oncogenes.

Loss of function mutations (*brake*) affect the genes that suppress growth or genes that drive the process of apoptosis.

Tumour suppressor genes inhibit the cell cycle. If their function is affected, then the cell cycle proceeds without inhibition. Fortunately, they act like a recessive gene, in that the effect is only manifest when both alleles of a chromosome are affected.

Oncogenes

Proto-oncogenes are genes that promote cell growth.

Oncogenes are 'rogue' proto-oncogenes because they have mutated. Their role is to continue to promote growth just like stepping down on the accelerator pedal in a car. These are more often acquired than inherited. The mutations that cause the proto-oncogene to become a 'rogue' are normally DNA duplication such as ABCDE to ABBCDE or rearrangement ABCDE to BACDE.

Inflammation

Inflammation is related to malignancy. It may be either the cause or the effect, but we are beginning to glean more into this aspect of malignant growth. Obesity causes chronic inflammation and is associated with increased malignancy.

Examples of inflammation and cancers are:
- *H. pylori* infections leading to chronic inflammation causing gastric cancers
- Bowel cancer and inflammatory bowel disease
- HPV and chronic cervicitis leading to cervical cancer
- Tobacco and lung inflammation leading to lung cancer

Equally, induced inflammation of the bladder with *Mycobacterium bovis* is a treatment for squamous cancers of the bladder.

Immune system

Cancer cells seem to evade detection by the innate and the adaptive immune system. But how? If only the cancer cells could be detected earlier by the dendritic cell, (Volume 1 of Snippets) then many cancers can be prevented at the outset. The immune surveillance system protects against many cancers. With each human being having more than 40 trillion cells, mutations occur almost daily in all. These are identified and rectified as long as the system works effectively. These are current areas of interest. A paradigm shift is occurring in the treatment of cancers with the advent of immunotherapy, immune modulation, and vaccination.

Immune checkpoint inhibitors that enable the T cell to recognise and destroy cancer cells are being studied with varying degrees of success. Monoclonal antibody treatment as in the treatment of HER2 positive breast cancers are enabling more patients to survive for longer than with traditional therapy. Targeted therapy such as CAR T-cell therapy for specific individuals and vaccination of certain tumours are being evaluated and will be discussed along with immunotherapy.

Section 5: Modes of therapy

Traditional management of cancers

Surgery was the cornerstone of treatment of cancers with the other modalities being used to contain cancers. With greater knowledge of cancer growth and spread and the realisation that cancer is a systemic disease, it became clear that other modalities of treatment may have increasingly more significant roles. Traditionally, the treatments focussed on:

- Surgery
- Radiotherapy
- Chemotherapy
- Hormone therapy

Immunotherapy surgery

"What remains in diseases after the crisis is apt to produce relapses"

—(Hippocrates)

Surgical resections for treatment are classified as being:

- Curative
- Palliative

It was presumed for many years that cancer progressed linearly from the site of origin to the lymph nodes and then to the blood stream and elsewhere in the body. It is now believed that cancers can be of the metastasising or the non-metastasising variety. The metastasis may, thus, occur in some unlucky patients even when the cancer is very tiny. In some patients where the cancer is detected early and there is no evidence of spread, a curative resection can be achieved.

In others, surgery is palliative and useful in controlling the local manifestations of the disease making the patient more comfortable. Death may occur due to effect of metastasis or nutritional depletion. Many patients with distant spread can be treated without resorting to invasive surgery but with some form of radiological or endoscopic intervention that *improves the quality of life without providing cure.*

Methods of spread

The cancer spreads by:

- Contiguity
- Lymphatics
- Blood stream

As tissues grow, they tend to invade surrounding tissues and involve neighbouring tissue.

As most of the tissues are well perfused with lymphatics and blood vessels it is logical to assume that the lymphatics and the blood stream are progressively involved. The sequence of this involvement is not clear but assumes that as the tumour increases in size it first invades the lymphatics and then progresses to other areas of the body by spreading through the blood stream. This model may not always be applicable as there are situations where the tumours metastasise through the blood stream even at the outset.

Surgery for confirmation of diagnosis

Surgery of one form or another is currently needed to confirm the diagnosis of malignancy. The biopsy or removal of tissue for histological scrutiny is the most common method of establishing the diagnosis.

Liquid biopsy tests are currently being assessed. These detect free floating DNA of tumour cells in blood.

Liquid biopsy tests

These are promising innovations in early cancer detection. They aim to detect circulating tumour DNA – ctDNA, and other biomarkers earlier and less invasively than other methods. At present false positives and false negatives are being studied.

Galleri test: This test may obviate the need for tissue sampling to confirm disease. It identifies DNA from cancer cells in the blood stream. This is being tested in the National Health Service in England on 1,65,000 people. The results are inconclusive but this is a step in screening for cancers in the population. It could be a game changer if tests such as these are able to predict the presence of cancer in asymptomatic patients. Early detection of the disease will save lives.

Shield test: A blood test for primary screening for colorectal cancer seems promising. The test, called, 'Shield' detects free cell DNA in blood. In a limited study, it detected 83% of patients who had a confirmed diagnosis of colorectal cancer. The sensitivity, however, was only 13% specific for polyps. It may be an adjunct to screening like the 'Faecal Immunochemical Test (*FIT*).

Surgical biopsy: This is of four types as follows:

1. Shave biopsy
2. Punch biopsy
3. Incisional biopsy
4. Excisional biopsy

Fine needle cytology or FNAC: Malignant cells tend not to stick to each other and as such are likely to be dislodged which gentle vibration of a needle or a spatula. *Papanicolaou* showed this to be feasible when he sampled cervical tissue in the presence of cervicitis. He noted the presence of malignant cells. This is the well-known 'Pap smear'. It is now possible to sample suspected malignant lesions and obtain cells that can be examined by the cytopathologist and assessed for the presence of malignancy.

Interventional surgery

In the *early evolution* of surgical management, the principle was *'cut more, cure more.'* For instance, with breast cancer, very mutilating surgery was carried out with a view to providing excision of all cancerous tissue. The disappointment became obvious when patients died of further cancer even after the most mutilating of operations where the entire chest wall was cleared of all the muscles and wounds left to heal by second intention. People did not live longer because of the *'radical'* surgery that eradicated the *'roots'* of cancer. The realisation dawned when follow-up after surgery showed that survival was not dependent on the radicality of the initial surgery.

Less surgery was as good as more and perhaps less was better because the mutilation was less.

It became clear that *surgery was best at delivering loco-regional control* but not necessarily cure in all patients with cancer.

The so-called *'adjuvant' therapy* with drugs would soon become the mainstay of treatment after debulking most of the cancer with a primary operation.

Radiotherapy

It is useful for:

- Cure of the disease (early stage)
- Control of the disease
- Control of symptoms (late stage)

Following surgery an effective modality of treatment of cancers is radiotherapy. This can be used for early tumours as well as for advanced tumours.

Radiotherapy works by damaging the DNA interfering with the process of replication and growth that is uncontrolled in malignant cells. Unlike chemotherapy, the effects of radiotherapy are very localised.

Types of radiotherapy

External beam radiotherapy

- *Conformal radiotherapy* which requires the use of CT scan to get a three-dimensional (3D) image also called 3D conformal radiotherapy or 3D-CRT.
- *Proton beam therapy* using protons rather than X-rays. This limits the damage to the surrounding tissue.
- *Stereotactic radiotherapy* delivers a high dose of radiotherapy to a very small area of the tumour. It requires cooperation of the patient as the patient must remain still to enable localisation. The treatment may be a single dose or more than one dose.

Internal beam radiotherapy: This includes brachy therapy where radiotherapy needles are inserted into the tissue for a short period of time such as in recurrent cervical and rectal cancers.

Histotripsy: This is a new non-invasive cancer treatment that uses focussed high intensity ultrasound that is directed towards the tumour. This creates bubble clouds from naturally occurring gases in the tissues. These bubbles form and collapse rapidly creating mechanical forces that destroys cells. It is being trialled in the UK from 2020 and trials show promise with potential for treatment of liver and kidney tumours initially.

Chemotherapy

After early attempts with nitrogen mustard and other agents, the first successful chemotherapy albeit for a transient and brief remission was with methotrexate. It, however, established the principle that cancers can be treated with drugs. These drugs are cytotoxic and they act on the cell cycle of all cells without discrimination of the cancer and normal cells. Most of the side effects are due to the effect of these cytotoxic agents on normal cells. Normal cells recover and, thus, the side effects settle over time.

Classification of chemotherapeutic agents

- *Alkylating agents* damage the DNA and act on all aspects of the cell cycle. Examples are carboplatin, cisplatin, cyclophosphamide, busulphan, melphalan, and thiotepa. Nitrosoureas are alkylating drugs that can cross the blood–brain barrier.
- *Antimetabolites* interfere with the DNA, RNA production and are useful in the treatment of leukaemia, breast, ovary and colon cancers. Examples are 5-flurouracil (5-FU), capecitabine, methotrexate, and hydroxyurea.
- *Antitumour antibodies* act by blocking DNA replication. Examples are doxorubicin and epirubicin. They are cardiotoxic.
- *Topoisomerase inhibitors:* These are also called plant alkaloids. They inhibit topoisomerase, which normally helps the DNA strands to separate. Examples are irinotecan and etoposide.
- *Mitotic inhibitors* such as taxanes and vinca alkaloids stop cell division. Examples are paclitaxel and vincristine.
- *Corticosteroids:* They are commonly used alongside chemotherapy.

Hormone therapy

Used commonly in the management of breast and prostate cancers.

Immuno therapy

Newer modalities targeted cancer therapies:

- *Monoclonal antibody therapy:* These are antibodies that are produced against targeted antigens on the surface of cancer cells. They can be used to:
  - *Block* growth
  - *Target* cancer cells
  - *Deliver* chemotherapy

Trastuzumab (Herceptin) binds to HER2 receptors and blocks growth. Rituximab binds to CD20 and enables the immune system to target the cancer cells.

These drugs have several side effects and in some can lead to capillary leak syndrome and multi organ failure. Skin reactions and infections are also common along with chills and flu-like symptoms.

- *CDK4/6* inhibitors
- *PIK3CA* inhibitors
- *mTOR* inhibitors
- *Epidermal growth factor receptor (EGFR)blocking agents:* The EGFRs are proteins that are found on the surface of normal cells. They are involved in the process of cell division. Some epithelial cancers, such as breast, colorectal, lungs, and ovaries have an over expression of EGFR leading to greater proliferation and poorer survival. EGFR inhibitors, such as cetuximab and erlotinib, are being used to treat EGFR expressing tumours. The relationship between increased expression of EGFR and survival is still being studied.

Immunotherapy harnesses the power of the immune system to seek and destroy cancer cells. Further progress in Immunotherapy over the last decade has enabled the development of CAR-T cell therapy, check point inhibitors, and cancer vaccines.

- *Cell therapy:* Chimeric antigen receptor T cells or CAR-T therapy. T cells are taken from an individual patient (autologous) or from a healthy donor (allogenic), cultured and genetically engineered to give them the ability to target specific antigens on the cancer cells. On binding to these antigens, the CAR-T cells become activated, proliferate, and become cytotoxic. The term Chimera is derived from Greek mythology where Chimera is a monster with a Goat's body but a lion's head and a serpent tail. In this context it is an engineered T cell that include structures it does not naturally have. Growing a patient's T cells and altering them takes time and is targeted for an individual patient.
- *Immune checkpoint inhibitors:* The immune check points are cell surface receptor – ligand (a signalling molecule) pairs found on tumour cells, T cells and antigen-presenting cells such as the dendritic cell. They must be distinguished from cell cycle checkpoint inhibitors that act on intracellular proteins that control cell division

Feature	**Cell cycle checkpoint inhibitors**	**Immune checkpoint inhibitors**
Target	Intracellular proteins that control cell division	Immune receptors that regulate T cell activity
Site of action	Inside the tumour cell cycle	At the *immune synapse* between T cells and tumour cells or antigen presenting cells
Mechanism of action	Forces cancer cells with DNA damage into apoptosis	Tumour cells express PD-L1 (programmed death-ligand 1) to evade the immune system. PD-1/PD-L1 inhibitors such as Nivolumab, block this interaction and activates the T cells enabling it to fight the tumour cells. Memory cells are also formed for long term surveillance enabling durable remissions
Primary effect	Directly destroys or sensitises tumour cells to chemotherapy	Destroys tumour cells by empowering patients own immune system
Side effects	Myelosuppression	Immune related events such as colitis, hepatitis, thyroiditis, myocarditis and skin rash
Usage	Tumours with defects in DNA, e.g. P53 loss, BRCA mutations	Tumours with immune visibility MSI -H, high PD-L1, etc.

The activation of the T cells to seek and destroy the malignant cells works as an extrinsic system. This system works even when P53 the guardian of the genome is mutated providing a different mechanism of control of malignancy.

Prognosis and recovery are multifactorial

They depend on:

- Patient's age
- Comorbidity
- Size of the tumour

- Grade of tumour which indicates rate of mitosis
- Stage which indicates distant spread to nodes or other locations
- Genetic propensity and mutations

Section 6: The TNM system

TNM system of staging cancer (**Figures 5 and 6**) is an accepted international standard for the classification of malignant tumour based on:

- T: Size of the primary Tumour. How large?
- N: Nodal status of the regional nodes. How many?
- M: Metastatic deposits. Where and how far? Extent of spread to other parts of the body such as lungs, liver and bones, etc.

It is assumed that tumours increase in size over time and then they spread to loco-regional nodes and subsequently to other parts of the body. This assumption may not always be true. Some types of cancers tend to metastasise from the outset. The causes for this are not yet clear but excluding that cohort, the TNM model is a recognised way of prognostication for all cancers.

TNM for breast cancer: The previous system of staging from 1 to 4 has been superseded by the TNM system for all cancers.

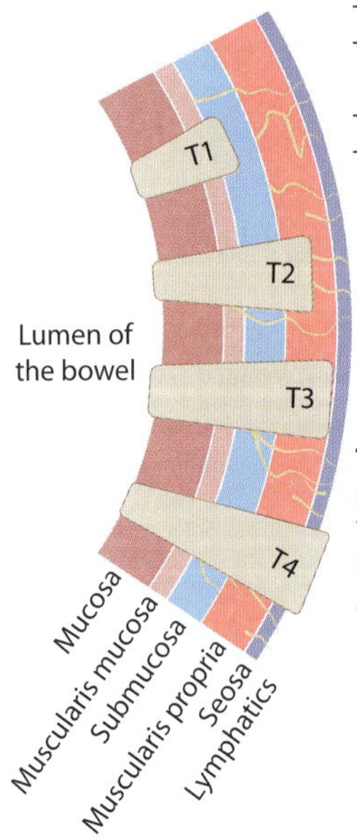

T1: Penetrates mucosa and submucosa
T2: Extends up to muscular layer-muscularis propria
T3: Extends up to serosal layer
T4: Extends beyond serosa involves adjacent tissue/organs

N0: No nodes involved
N1: 1–3 nodes involved
N2: >4 nodes invoved

M0: No metastasis detected
M1: Metastasis present

Tx, Nx, Mx: x denotes stage not assessed
Y: Prefix indicates staging has been affected by adjuvant chemo- or radiotherapy

TME: 'Total mesorectal excision' is the term used for rectal cancer resection
CRM: 'Circumferential resection margin': This must be differentiated from distal and proximal resection margins

Duke's staging remains in usage
Dukes A: Tumour extends to submucosa
Dukes B: Tumour extends through the wall
Dukes C: Tumour involves nodes
Duke did not stage metastasis

Figure 5 Staging of colorectal cancer.

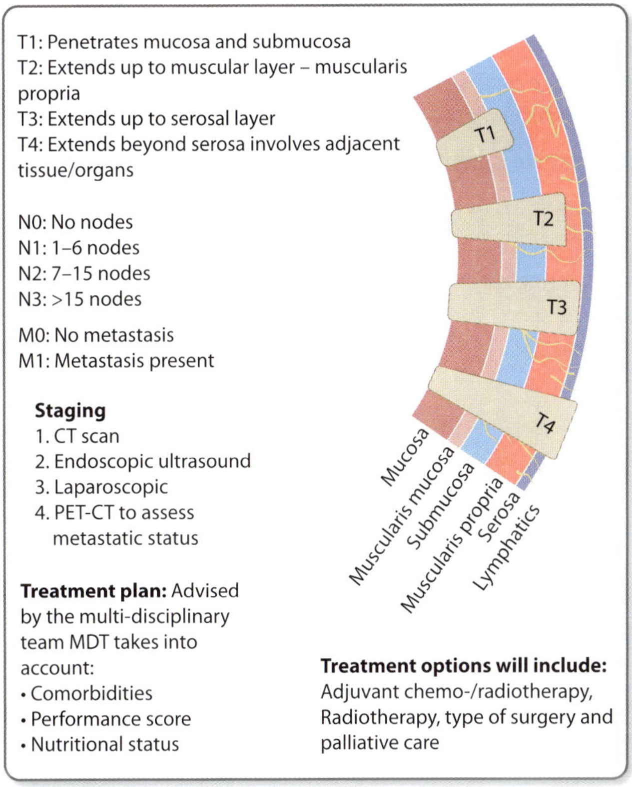

Figure 6: Staging of gastro-oesophageal cancer.

Tumour:

TX: Primary tumour is not assessed.

T0: There is no evidence of the primary tumour.

Tis: Ductal carcinoma (intraduct) in situ or Paget's disease of the breast with no related invasive tumour.

T1: Original tumour diameter is ≤2 cm.

T2: Original tumour diameter is between 2 and 5 cm.

T3: Original tumour diameter is >5 cm.

T4: Original tumour has invaded other organs, like the chest wall or skin.

Nodes:

NX: Lymph nodes not assessed.

N0: There is no spread to nearby lymph nodes.

N1: Cancer has spread to fewer than three lymph nodes in the axilla or to any number of lymph nodes of the internal mammary chain of lymph nodes.

N2: Cancer has spread to between 4 and 9 lymph nodes of the underarm.

N3: Cancer has spread to >10 lymph nodes of the axilla, and to lymph nodes under the clavicle.

Metastasis:

M0: No distant spread detected in the body via imaging tests.

M1: Spread detected in one or more distant areas of the body, such as the bones or brain.

In addition to TNM, the *hormonal receptor status of the breast cancer* is also added in the final analysis. These include the presence or absence of *oestrogen or progesterone receptors* and presence or absence of *human epidermal growth factor receptor 2 – HER2.*

Estrogen receptor (ER) positive or negative is represented as:
- ER positive
- ER negative

Progesterone receptor (PR) positive or negative as:
- PR positive
- PR negative

HER2 status as:
- HER2 positive
- HER2 negative

Grading of the cancer as to how malignant the cells are as per WHO grading (G): Graded from 1 to 3 based on cytological assessment
- Grade 1: Low grade
- Grade 2: Intermediate grade
- Grade 3: High grade

Section 7: Multidisciplinary teams and causes of death in patients with cancer

Multidisciplinary teams are a group of healthcare workers from various disciplines who contribute to the provision of healthcare for an individual patient. In regard to the management of cancers, the team may include surgeons, physicians, radiologists, oncologists, histopathologists, nurses and co-ordinators. Teams adhere to the recommendations of the multidisciplinary team for the management of a particular patient, but it must be stated that these are essentially for the best guidance. Variations in the final delivery of care is still possible and is determined by the discussions between the patient and his carers.

The patient journey starts from initial presentation and standardises delivery of an acceptable level of care.
- Presentation to primary care
- Referral to secondary care based on referral criteria
- Assessment of patient
- Organisation of investigations
- Review of patient with results
- Communication with patient and carers
- Discussion of all available information at a multidisciplinary team meeting
- Final decision as to the treatment options which will include curative and palliative care:
  - Non-surgical management
  - Surgical management
  - Chemotherapy

- Radiotherapy, and
- Palliative care
- Implementation following discussion with patient and carers
- Post-treatment follow-up plan

Pathway of care of the cancer patient

Care pathways are a way of standardising best practice in the management of a particular condition suffered by the patient. These pathways also referred to as integrated care pathways act as a guide to the management of patients. It permits auditing of results and allows for the entire care journey of an individual patient to be set out at the outset.

The patient journey starts at the point of referral from the primary care to the secondary care sector. The pathway sets out the timelines for care culminating in a co-ordinated multidisciplinary meeting when the final decision for the management of a patient with cancer can be set out. This process of planning the management of all cancer patients permits standardisation.

Causes of death in cancer patients

JL Ambrus et al. analysed the causes of death based on clinical and pathologic reports of 506 cases in the Roswell Park Memorial Institute and Hospital.
The causes were identified as:

- *Infection (36%):* It was a major contributory factor in other cancer related deaths.
- *Respiratory failure* (19%) due to various causes (including aspiration)
- *Haemorrhagic and thromboembolic phenomena* (18%)
- *Organ invasion* (10%) by neoplastic cells including hepatic failure
- *Cardiovascular* (7%) insufficiency
- *Cachexia* (1%)

Intercurrent infections are the most common cause of death in patients dying of malignancy.

Rapid death when it occurs is due to haemorrhage from infiltration of major vessels.

Nutritional depletion and poor immunological system contribute to death from infections.

Section 8: Appendix – significant papers and information

William Halsted in his presentation to the American Surgical Association in May 1907 concluded that the following factors affected the ultimate results in the management of cancers.

- The variety of the cancer
- Time elapsed since its initial appearance
- The degree of outlying involvement
- The thoroughness of the operation

He set out the following surgical principles.

- Handle tissues gently.
- Maximise haemostasis.
- Retain vascularity of tissues.
- Follow asepsis – he used antiseptics and surgical gloves.

- Reduce tension when apposing edges.
- Do not leave a blind space.

Radiotherapy

Wilhelm Conrad Röntgen discovered X-rays in 1895 and contributed vastly to the management of malignancies. *Antoine Henri Becquerel* started to study the phenomenon of radioactivity and its sources at about the same time. In 1898, *Maria Sklodowska-Curie* and her husband *Pierre Curie* discovered the *radium* as a source of radiation. And, subsequently, along with Becquerel Maria reported the physiological effects of radiotherapy. Initially, only superficial radiation was used to treat some skin cancers, but *Coolidge* developed a machine that could be used to deliver radiation to deeper tissues in early 20th century.

Fractionated doses rather than single doses were shown to treat cancer better in the 1920s followed by the realisation for *radiation protection* later in that decade.

Robert McWhirter, a radiotherapist from Edinburgh, introduced a system of radiotherapy for breast cancer in 1948, that showed that breast cancer could be treated without radical mastectomy when combined with his system of radiotherapy. He showed that less mutilating surgery combined with radiotherapy could deliver similar results.

Norman Nigro, in 1974, published a study that showed that combining 5-F and mitomycin-C with external beam radiotherapy for anal cancers, resulted in a complete response. This study reduced the need for radical abdomino-perineal resection for anal canal cancers.

In 2004, *Habr-Gama* from the University of Sao Paulo, Brazil, published the results of chemo-radiotherapy (CRT) for resectable rectal cancers. In a study of 265 patients, 71 patients had a complete response. He concluded that stage 0 rectal cancer disease is associated with excellent long-term results irrespective of treatment strategy. Surgical resection may not lead to improved outcome in this situation and may be associated with high rates of temporary or definitive stoma construction and unnecessary morbidity and mortality rates.

Chemotherapy

In 1948, *Sidney Faber,* a pathologist working at Harvard Medical school successfully induced remission in childhood leukaemia using analogues of folic acid developed by *Yellapragada Subbarao* who was working with Lederle. Subbarao is also co-credited with the *discovery of ATP.* He was working on folic acid and its analogues aminopterin and *amethopterin* (methotrexate). Folic acid had been discovered by *Lucy Wills* in 1937 while working in *Bombay* (now Mumbai) as being crucial in preventing megaloblastic anaemia of pregnancy in India; but treating childhood leukaemia with it worsened the condition.

An analogue of folic acid amethopterin was noted to be antagonistic to folic acid. Subbarao arranged to deliver it to Faber who was exploring the possibility of treating childhood leukaemia with a folic acid antagonist as folic acid is required for the growth of white and red blood cells. If one can block its action, Faber felt leukaemia could be controlled. The first known remission although not long lasting was produced with amethopterin establishing the principle of chemotherapy as an acceptable treatment for cancers. *Methotrexate*is still in use today. Writing in the April 1950 issue of Argosy, Doron K. Antrim observed, "You've probably never heard of Dr. Yellapragada Subbarao. Yet because he lived, you may be alive and are well today. Because he lived, you may live longer."

Chapter 3

Breast disease

Srinivasan Ravi

Section 1: Breast lumps (Figures 1 to 3)

The breast overlies the pectoralis major and minor muscles. The minor is deeper and intimately related to the axillary vessels and the lymphatic chain. There are over 20 glands interspersed between fatty tissue that make up the breast. These drain to the nipple. 60% of the glands are located in the upper outer quadrant of the breast and hence breast lumps are more common in this region

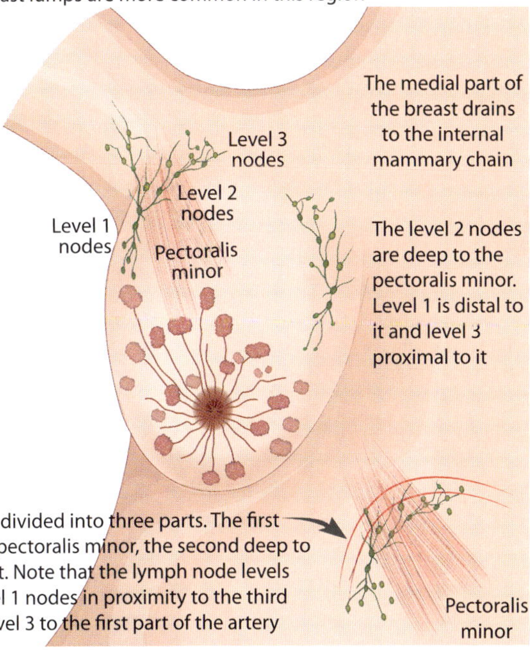

Figure 1 Basic anatomy of breast.

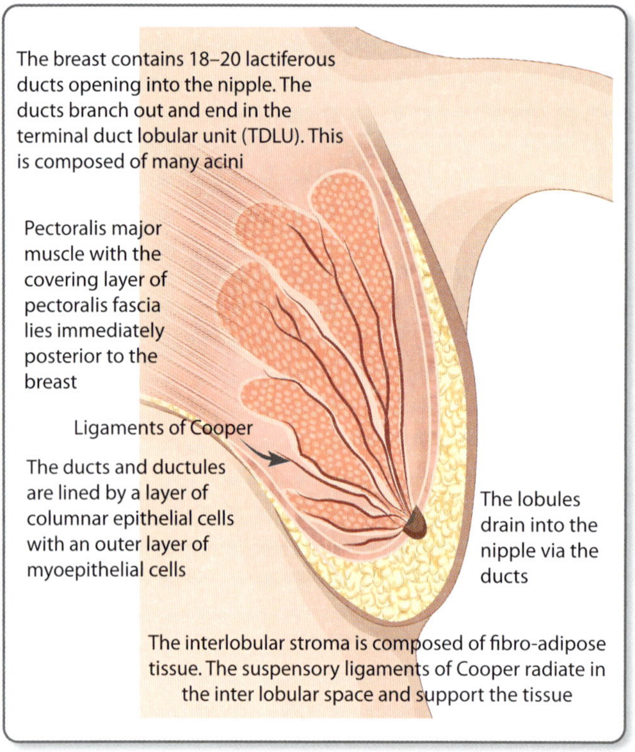

Figure 2 Structure of the breast.

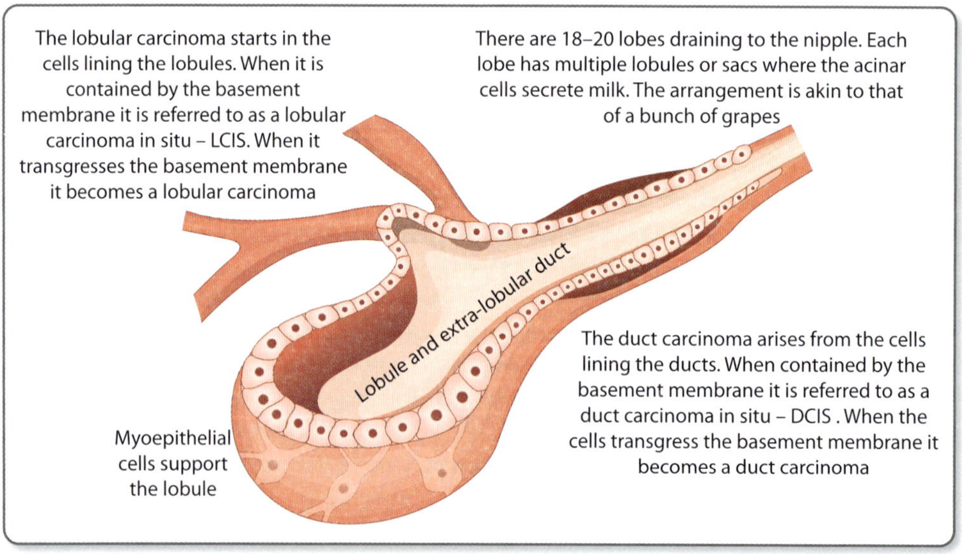

Figure 3 The lobule of the breast.

- Benign disease is more common than malignant disease.
- Malignant breast disease is mostly of ductal or lobular origin and can be in-situ or invasive.
- Breast lumps can be due to:
  - *Fibroadenoma* a benign tumour common in young girls and young women. It is typically very mobile and because of its mobility it slips and moves away from the palpating hand. It is referred to as a 'breast mouse'.
  - *Fibrocystic disease* a common cause that classically presents with multiple cysts and areas of thickening and represents a benign spectrum of disease.
  - *Subareolar lumps* that can be due to duct ectasia or dilated ducts. Rarely, they may be due to a duct papilloma or carcinoma.
  - *Fat necrosis* which may arise following recognised or unrecognised trauma. They may mimic a breast cancer.
  - *Breast abscess* which can present acutely as a painful and warm lump.
  - *Phyllodes tumours* (from leaflike in Greek) arise from connective tissue of the breast.
  - *Gynaecomastia* in males
  - *Breast cancer* which typically has a firmer consistency and may be fixed to the skin, with tethering of the skin or deeper structures such as the pectoralis major muscle.

Nipple discharge

Nipple discharge is not uncommon in women and occasional discharge is noted by many women from time to time.
It can be:

- Clear
- Greenish
- Purulent
- Bloody

Discharges from the nipple need attention if:

- It is persistent from the same breast.
- If it is bloody.
- If it is foul smelling.
- If the woman is over 50 years of age.
- If it occurs in a male.

Fibroadenoma

They are common in the age group of 20–30 years but may occur in teenagers and elderly women on hormone replacement.

A confirmatory cytology along with either ultrasound or mammographic imaging may be needed.

In the very young a non-operative management may be followed but, in most women, surgical excision and histological confirmation will be necessary.

Fibrocystic disease

These patients present with a pain-free lump that sometimes seems to occur overnight. When the cysts are due to blocked ducts, they may feel hard due to the tension on the wall of the cyst from fluid within akin to a tense water-filled balloon. Although they cause a lot of anxiety, they are seldom malignant.

Imaging with ultrasound followed by aspiration and reassurance suffices in most.

When the aspirate is clear, there is seldom a need for confirmatory cytology although it may be needed to allay the anxiety; however, if the aspirate is bloody, cytology is needed.

On aspiration most of these cysts disappear and if they recur further aspiration may be needed.

ANDI (aberrations of normal development and involution) is a modern framework that reclassifies most benign breast conditions such as fibrocystic disease as normal variations of breast tissue due to hormones rather than actual disease. It encompasses, cysts, fibrosis and even fibroadenomas as part of the nromal hormonal cycle and ageing process.

Subareolar lumps

These are noted in the areolar tissue and do not involve the nipple. Commonly they are due to the dilatation of the ducts with retained collection sometimes leading to tethering.

When due to *duct papilloma* they may present with a bloody discharge and will need identification and excision of the appropriate duct.

Fat necrosis

This can mimic a breast cancer. It is due to trauma and sometimes follows surgical lumpectomy or biopsy. Since the necrosis pulls in the fatty tissue around it, very many of these lumps may feel hard. To confirm the diagnosis, they will need cytology or in some even an excision biopsy.

Breast abscess

Presentation is normally acute and may occur in lactating women. The lump is tender and may in a few be accompanied by fever. If the exhibition of antibiotics fails to promote resolution they will need aspiration, sometimes multiple times or incision and drainage.

Phyllodes tumour

The diagnosis is generally made histologically as they may present like a fibroadenoma. Sometimes they grow rapidly and involve the whole breast.

These are almost always benign with about *10% of the tumours undergoing malignant change to a sarcoma* as the origin is the connective tissue and not ducts.

In most, a lumpectomy should suffice but a mastectomy may be needed in a few when the tumour is very big.

Gynaecomastia

This is due to enlargement of breast tissue in men. It occurs due to *hormonal imbalance* between testosterone and oestrogen.

The imbalance can occur during puberty and in men as they age and the testosterone level decreases.

It can occur in infants due to the high levels of *maternal oestrogen. Medications* such as cimetidine and proton pump inhibitors (PPIs), spironolactone, 5-α reductase blockers, verapamil, nifedipine, opioids and drugs for HIV have all been implicated.

Section 2: Breast cancer – pathology

Carcinoma of the breast is the most common cancer worldwide accounting for >2 million new cases a year. Breast cancer essentially comprises two main types – lobular (arising from the lobules) and ductal (arising from the ducts). When the neoplastic change is confined by the basement membrane, the cancers are called *in situ* as opposed to *invasive* lesions. Other histologically different cancers are <10% of all breast cancers.

Pathology

Common types of neoplastic lesions are:

In situ neoplasia

- Duct carcinoma in situ – DCIS
- Lobular carcinoma in situ – LCIS

Invasive carcinoma

- Duct carcinoma
- Lobular carcinoma

Duct carcinoma

- Constitute about 75% of all breast cancers.
- Have a propensity to multicentricity.
- Show up as microcalcifications/skin thickening on mammograms and, hence, are screen detectable.

Lobular carcinoma

- Have a propensity to bilaterality.
- May be invisible on mammograms.
- May not be detected on screening.
- Constitute about 15% of breast cancers.

DCIS – duct carcinoma in situ

- This is considered to be a precursor of breast cancer.
- It is a preinvasive breast cancer (IBC) (*Cancer research, UK*).
- Can be low, intermediate or high-grade tumours.
- Low-grade tumours may be difficult to distinguish from dysplasia.
- High-grade tumours can undergo change to invasive cancer.

LCIS – lobular carcinoma in situ

- This is a risk factor for cancer.
- It is not yet a cancer.
- LCIS has an increased risk of turning to invasive cancer.

- This risk is thought to be approximately 20% (*Mayo Clinic*).
- LCIS can be invisible on mammograms.
- It is commonly an incidental finding.

Notes:

1. Invasive ductal carcinoma is now termed as 'invasive carcinoma of no special type (NST).'
2. Lobular carcinoma in situ (LCIS) is now termed as 'lobular neoplasia,' an umbrella term that incorporates both LCIS (as previously known) and atypical lobular hyperplasia.
3. Despite commonly used traditional morphological classification of breast cancer as ductal (arising from the ductal system) and lobular (arising from the lobule), the current evidence shows that most benign and malignant breast lesions originate from the same anatomical compartment, the *terminal ductal lobular units (TDLU).*

Other types of breast cancers:

- *Medullary carcinoma* – afflicts younger patients and has a high prevalence of *BRCA1* gene mutation.
- *Mucinous carcinoma* – contains extracellular mucin and is more common in the elderly.
- *Inflammatory breast cancer* in younger women tends to progress rapidly and has a poorer prognosis.
- *Phyllodes tumours* with malignant transformation
- *Paget's disease* with duct carcinoma characterised by the presence of large Paget cells with hyperchromatic nuclei. In these the nipple is always involved.
- *Tubular and papillary carcinoma*

Section 3: Risk factors and presentation

Risk factors for breast cancer

- Female
- Early menarche
- Late menopause
- Nulliparous
- Previous cancer in one breast
- Previous in situ cancer
- Family history
- *BRCA* (*BR*east *CA*ncer)-*1* and -*2* genes
- Obesity
- Alcohol intake more than normal
- Hormone replacement therapy (HRT) oestrogen/progesterone combination is worse that oestrogen alone but all HRT increases risk (2019).
- Previous radiotherapy to chest

Risk reduction for breast cancer

- Increased breast awareness – with self-examination
- Breast screening

- Maintaining ideal body weight with lifestyle changes as necessary
- Drinking alcohol in moderation
- Modulating use of post-menopausal HRT

Presentation of breast cancer

- Mass or lump
- Ulcerating lesion
- Mammogram detection
- Palpable metastatic axillary node
- Inverted or retracted nipple

Referral criteria: Men/Women – NICE guidance

- 30 years or older with a breast lump that is not caused by anything else.
- 50 years or older with changes to nipple such as discharge from the nipple or nipple retraction or inversion.
- 30 years or older and have a lump in the axilla that is not thought to be due to skin problems.

Section 4: Investigations for breast lumps

Most patients, even those presenting with clinically benign disease, will need to be assessed and subjected to clinical, radiological, and cytological assessments.

The assessment and diagnosis are now standardised as per the NICE guidance and can be summarised as follows:

- On diagnosis of a suspected breast lump the patient is referred urgently to a specialist centre.
- *A triple assessment* is carried out and this involves:
  - *Clinical* assessment with history taking and full examination
  - *Radiological* assessment with mammogram and, if necessary, an ultrasound examination of the breast and axilla
  - *Cytological* (pathological) assessment with a fine needle aspiration cytology (FNAC) or a core biopsy – to get histology
- Grading (**Table 1**) is carried out and is similar for Palpation (*P*), Mammography (*M*), Cytology (*C*), Biopsy (*B*). The grading from 1 not malignant to 5 or malignant as follows:
  - P1 to P5 staging for palpation findings

Table 1 Grading: Breast lumps.

P1, M1, C1 and B1	Normal
P2, M2, C2 and B2	Benign
P3, M3, C3 and B3	Uncertain/Benign
P4, M4, C4 and B4	Possibly malignant
P5, M5, C5 and B5	Malignant

  - M1 to M5 staging for mammographic findings
  - U1 to U5 staging for ultrasound findings
  - C1 to C5 or B1 to B5 staging for cytology or biopsy findings
- On confirmation of malignancy, the patient is allocated a designated *specialist nurse.*
- *Receptor status:* The oestrogen receptor (ER), progesterone receptor (PR) and human epidermal growth factor receptor 2 (*HER2*) status of the tumour assessed
- *Genetic testing for BRCA* is offered when 'triple negative' for receptors and when there is a strong family history.
- *Ultrasound evaluation of the axilla* is needed for early invasive breast cancer (IBC). If abnormal lymph nodes are identified, ultrasoundguided needle sampling is done.
- *Additional breast imaging modalities* include MRI scan and tomosynthesis (CT scan of breast), with or without contrast.
- *Metastatic work-up* may entail CT chest, abdomen, pelvis, Technetium-99m (99mTc) bone scan, 18F-fluorodeoxyglucose (FDG) positron emission tomography (PET)-CT, and 18F-sodium fluoride (NaF) skeletal PET-CT.
- The findings are discussed at a *multidisciplinary team (MDT)* with oncologists, radiologists, pathologist, nurse specialists and surgeons.
- A *treatment plan* will be made out for each patient at the MDT.

Mammography

It is a low-dose X-ray of the breast involving breast compression between plates to get clear images.

- Mammography detects breast cancer by revealing abnormal patterns in breast tissue that differ from normal structures.
- *Specific signs on the mammogram image*:
  - *Masses or lumps*: Appear as dense, white areas compared to surrounding normal fat or glandular tissue, making it stand out.
  - *Microcalcifications*: Tiny deposits of calcium that show up as bright white specks. Certain patterns (clustered, irregular shapes) may suggest early cancer.
  - *Distorted architecture*: Cancer may pull or distort tissue, creating unusual shapes or asymmetry. Overlying skin may be thickened.
  - *Differences between breasts*: Comparing left and right breast images helps spot subtle changes.

TNM for breast cancer (Table 2)

TNM is the global standard for staging breast cancer based on tumour size, nodal spread and presence or absence of metastasis, as discussed in the chapter on Oncology. Current breast cancer staging American Joint Committee on Cancer (AJCC 8th Ed) goes beyond TNM to include prognostic factors such as grade, hormone receptor status and HER2 status.

Standard work-up

a. Confirm diagnosis of malignancy with cytology.

b. Confirm grade of malignancy.

Table 2 TNM for breast cancer.	
Tx	Primary tumour is not assessed.
T0	There is no evidence of the primary tumour
Tis	In situ ductal carcinoma/Paget's with no related tumour
T1	Original tumour 2 cm or less
T2	Original tumour between 2 and 5 cm
T3	Original tumour > 5 cm
T4	Original tumour has invaded adjacent tissue/organs
Nx	Lymph nodes not assessed
N0	No spread to lymph nodes
N1	• Involves three lymph nodes or less in axilla • Spread to any number of internal mammary chain
N2	Involves 4–9 axillary chain nodes
N3	Involves >10 axillary/subclavicular nodes
M0	No distant metastases detected on imaging
M1	Metastasis to one or more distant areas; brain, bones, etc.

c. Confirm nodal status.

d. Confirm hormonal status.

Hormonal receptor status

In addition to TNM (**Table 2**) the hormonal receptor status of the breast cancer is also added in the final analysis. These include the presence or absence of ER or PRs and presence or absence of *HER2*.

Oestrogen receptor positive or negative is represented as:

- ER positive
- ER negative

Progesterone receptor positive or negative as:

- PR positive
- PR negative
- *ER/PR is considered positive if* Allred score is 3–8 (out of *maximum* 8), or ≥1% of tumour cells demonstrate positive nuclear staining by immunohistochemistry.

Human epidermal growth factor receptor 2 status as:

- *HER2* positive
- *HER2* negative

Grading

Grading of the cancer as to how malignant the cells are as per WHO grading (G). This is graded from 1 to 3 based on cytological assessment.

- *Grade 1:* Low grade

- *Grade 2:* Intermediate grade
- *Grade 3:* High grade

The *Borders* grading of cytology as discussed earlier was subsequently changed by the WHO to grades 1 to 3 based on well-differentiated, moderately differentiated, and poorly differentiated cancers.

This is the basis for grading of FNAC in breast cancer to the five grades C1 to C5. C5 is clearly malignant and C1 is clearly not malignant.

Fine needle aspiration cytology is carried out under ultrasound imaging guidance. It is particularly useful for non-palpable lesions in symptomatic and screening populations.

Core biopsy (tissue diagnosis) is advantageous over FNAC, as it helps in:

- Distinguishing between in situ and invasive cancer
- Diagnosing type of cancer
- Assessing grade, receptor status and lympho-vascular invasion

Core biopsy can be performed under:

- *Ultrasound guidance:* This is most commonly used.
- *MRI guidance* when the lesion is only visible on MRI.
- *Stereotactic core biopsy* under mammographic guidance for microcalcifications and for mammographically detected lesions that are not clearly seen on ultrasound.

Prognostic factors

Prognostic factors are associated with probable course of the breast cancer (for example, disease-free survival, overall survival, etc.). The probability can be influenced by the treatment.

- Age and method of diagnosis (i.e. screening versus symptomatic)
- Size, type and grade of the primary – larger the original tumour size the poorer the prognosis
- Presence of comedo necrosis and focality
- Hormone receptor status when positive, the outcome is favourable.
- Resection margin
- *Lympho-vascular invasion:* Axillary nodal status - presence of more than four nodes has a poor prognosis.
- Tumour size response to neo-adjuvant systemic treatment

Prognostic Impact of Luminal classification of breast cancer

Luminal A and Luminal B are subtypes of breast cancers identified through immunohistochemistry markers including ER, PR, HER2 as well as the proliferation marker Ki-67 which defines the aggressiveness. Both are classified as hormone receptor-positive, but they differ in their molecular features, prognosis, and treatment approaches **(Table 3)**.

Predictive factors

Predictive factors are associated with the probability of the effect of a given therapy. Following are the common examples of predictive factors in breast cancer:

- ER/PR status
- *HER2* status

Table 3 The identification of breast cancer subtype is useful in the management.		
Feature	**Luminal A**	**Luminal B**
ER/PR status	Positive	Positive
HER2 status	Negative	Negative or Positive
Ki-67 proliferation	Low	High
Growth rate	Slow	Faster
Prognosis	Favourable	Less favourable
Treatment	Hormonal therapy	Hormonal therapy, chemotherapy, ± targeted therapy

Note:

- Luminal A cancers may be managed with hormonal therapy alone.
- Luminal B cancers, due to their higher risk of recurrence, often require more intensive treatment, which may include chemotherapy and HER2-targeted agents when applicable.

- Results of tumour genetic profiling test (e.g. EndoPredict, Oncotype DX Breast Recurrence Score and Prosigna)

Nottingham prognostic index (Table 4)

This is another prognostic tool to enable decision making and titrating treatment for every patient preventing over or under treatment. The Nottingham prognostic index (NPI) has been validated by many studies as a useful prognostic predictor in the management of breast cancer. It is based on the size of the tumour, the lymph nodal stage and the grade of malignancy.

Table 4 5-year survival prediction.	
Score	**5-year survival**
2.4 or less	93%
2.4–3.4	85%
3.4–5.4	70%
>5.4	50%

Source: Haybittle JL, Blamey RW, Elston CW, Johnson J, Doyle PJ, Campbell FC, et al. A prognostic index in primary breast cancer. Br J Cancer 1982; 45:361–366.

$$\text{NPI} = \text{maximum invasive cancer size (S)} \times 0.2 + \text{lymph node stage (LN} = 1, 2, \text{or } 3) + \text{histological grade (H} = 1, 2, \text{or } 3)$$

- S - Size in centimetres
- N -Nodal status. 0 nodes - 1, 1-3 - 2 and >3 - 3
- G Grading from 1 to 3

Section 5: Hormone receptor status

Breast cancer cells may have receptors on the surface of cells that are sensitive to oestrogen and progesterone.

When cells have the appropriate receptors, they are referred to as ER or PR positive (the American spelling 'estrogen receptor' is used for ER).

The presence of receptors indicates the sensitivity of the tumours to the hormones, oestrogen, or progesterone. If these can be blocked, the growth of cancer can be suppressed. Positive receptor status allows blocking with antioestrogens like tamoxifen and aromatase inhibitors like arimidex.

Genetic status

HER2 or human epidermal growth factor 2 is a gene that is present in all breast cells that make a recognisable protein that is located on the surface of cells; it assists growth. When *HER2* is mutated, a greater number of the cell surface protein is present; it enhances growth leading to cancers. When an increased amount of *HER2* protein is expressed, it is referred to as a *HER2* receptor positive cancer.

If the levels are normal, the cancer is graded HER2 negative.

Approximately 20% of breast cancers are *HER2* positive. *HER2* receptor positive tumours respond to treatment by blocking agents like herceptin.

Breast cancer genes – BRCA1 and -2 are present in approximately 5–10% of patients with breast cancer. If their presence is known, more careful monitoring or even prophylactic mastectomies may be a consideration. There may be other genes that are yet to be recognised. The author knows of a family with all the five sisters and their children with breast cancer but remain negative for the currently recognised genes.

Triple negative breast cancer

This type of cancer tests negative for all the three protein receptors present in cancer cells. These are:

1. Oestrogen
2. Progesterone
3. Human epidermal growth receptors (*HER2*)

Triple negative breast cancers (TNBC) are more common in:

- Women under 40 years of age
- Black women
- Women with *BRCA1*

The absence of receptors with which to bind means that hormone-blocking treatments are ineffective.

These are likely to benefit from:

- Chemotherapy
- Immunotherapy
- Surgery including mastectomy
- Radiation therapy
- Bisphosphonate treatment

Breast cancers can be multicentric a principle that was known even in the days of Halstead. It stands to reason that removing a lump alone as in a lumpectomy might leave other foci untreated. Treating the whole breast is mandatory in most cases; if a surgeon does not do a mastectomy and only removes the lump, the rest of the breast must also be treated; this is addressed by radiotherapy, hormone therapy or chemotherapy.

Section 6: Sentinel node biopsy

Sentinel (sentry) node is the first node in the axilla that may be involved by spread from the primary breast cancer. Sometimes there can be more than one node (National Institute of Health). Sentinel lymph node biopsy (SLNB) is based on the concept that the tumour spreads from the primary to the nodes and then elsewhere to the rest of the body – a concept proposed by Halstead!

In one trial, involving 5,611 women, researchers randomly assigned participants to receive just SLNB, or SLNB plus axillary lymph node dissection (ALND), after surgery. 3,989 women in the two groups whose sentinel lymph node(s) were negative for cancer were followed for an average of 8 years. The researchers found no differences in overall survival or disease-free survival between the two groups of women.

Source: Krag DN, Anderson SJ, Julian TB, Brown AM, Harlow SP, Ashikaga T, et al. Technical outcomes of sentinel-lymph-node resection and conventional axillary-lymph-node dissection in patients with clinically node-negative breast cancer: results from the NSABP B-32 randomised phase III trial. Lancet Oncol 2007; 8:881–888.

If the nodes are not involved, there is little point in subjecting the patient to a more major procedure such as axillary lymph node dissection – ALND.

Sentinel lymph node (SLN) biopsy is a tool for lymph node mapping for the patient with *early-stage invasive breast cancer (IBC) and a clinically negative axilla.*

This assesses the involvement of axillary nodes by instilling a *radioisotope and blue dye* in the breast around the primary tumour.

SLNs are successfully *localised by a hand-held Geiger counter* that picks up the radiation if there is spread to the axilla.

If radiation is detected in the axilla, then the axilla is dissected and the node localised by the presence of the staining induced by the dye that is instilled along with the radioisotope.

Sentinel lymph node dissection (SLND) can then be carried out.

SNB (sentinel node biopsy) can also be performed by using alternative techniques, such as:

- Iron oxide particles (Magtrace tracer)
- Indocyanine green (ICG) dye

SLNB obviates the need for axillary dissection and reduces complications such as lymphoedema in many patients.

Section 7: Survival after breast cancer (Table 5)

It is a sobering thought to reflect on the fact that even tumours as small as 0.5 cm in size may have micro-metastasis in the axillary glands and many patients with curative resection may yet die of metastasis in the future. This is due to biological predeterminism – a tumour's growth is predicted by its innate histological character.

When a breast cancer reaches 1 cm in size, it has undergone 30 doublings. The doubling time is the time it takes for one cell to become two. The doubling time for breast cancer is approximately 180 days (discussed in the chapter on Oncology).

(Cancer Medicine: "Open access review. Has tumour doubling time in breast cancer changed over the past 80 years? A systematic review).

Table 5 Survival after breast cancer.

Alive at 5 years	80%
Alive at 10 years	75%
Alive at 20 years	65% (two-thirds)

Note: Early cancers under 2 cm size: 90% alive at 5 years.
Source: 2019 Gov.UK . The current changes in chemotherapy and monoclonal therapy will cause a paradigm shift in the survival.

At 40 doublings, the cancer normally kills the host! This is true of all malignancies as they outstrip the ability of the host to provide nutrition. It is very Malthusian in its manifestation!

Surgical treatment of breast cancer is carried out to control loco-regional disease spread. Surgery does not affect the systemic spread of the disease unless it is picked up very early, by screening or good luck, before the spread has occurred.

Systemic disease is best treated with chemotherapy or hormonal manipulation.

Section 8: Screening for breast cancer

Sir Muir Gray chair of the UK National Screening Committee said in his keynote speech on videos worth watching – *Gov.UK that*

"All screening programmes do harm. This is from the book we wrote on the basis of our experience in screening called 'Screening: evidence and practice.' The second sentence says some do good as well and of these some do more good than harm at a reasonable cost".

Around 2,116,588 women were screened by the UK NHS Breast Screening Programme (NHSBSP) between 1 April 2008 and 31 March 2009.

17,045 cancers were detected (*8.1 per 1,000 women screened*). Of which 13,532 (79%) were invasive (*6.4 per 1,000 women screened*).

The origins of breast cancer screening

Women aged 40–64 years were selected from members in the Health Insurance Plan (HIP) of Greater New York. They were randomly assigned to study and control groups.

Study group women were invited for screening, an initial examination, and three annual re-examinations. Screening consisted of mammography (cephalocaudal and lateral views of each breast) and clinical examination of breasts. Breast cancer and mortality from breast cancer were examined by treatment group (study vs. control) and by entry-age subgroup.

By the end of 18 years from entry, the study group had about a 25% lower breast cancer mortality among women aged 40–49 years and 50–59 years at time of entry than did the control group.

This was the basis for the introduction of breast screening programmes in many parts of the world.

Many have criticised screening programmes in general because the results of screening programmes seem to be biased due to various factors, in particular 'lead time' bias. Others argue that there will perhaps be no major impact of screening for the population as a whole if people presented with symptoms and were then treated appropriately. One must know about the pros and cons of false positives and false negatives to have enlightened discussions with patients.

The pickup rate of cancers is comparatively small for the cost of screening.

The impact for the patient who has early detection and treatment, however, is very considerable.

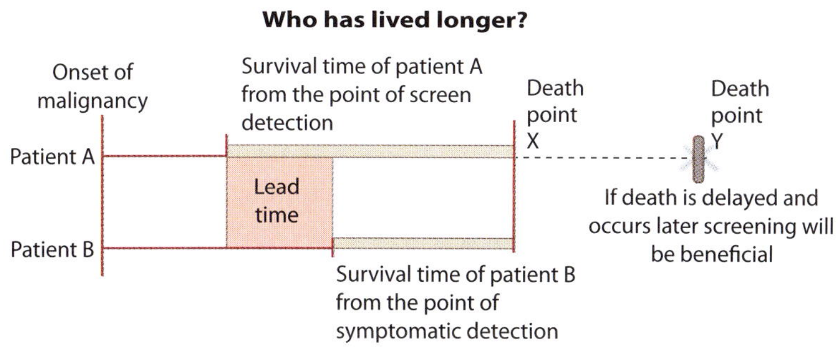

If the patients A and B die at the same point in time patient A would, as a result of screening be deemed to have lived longer because of the lead time bias. This would not be a true increase in survival time. If, however, patient A dies at Y instead of X, the patient would have truly lived longer because of earlier detection and treatment

Figure 4 Lead time bias.

Data from the All-Breast Cancer Report show that 27% of all breast cancers were screen-detected.

Lead time bias (Figure 4)

Lead time is the time interval between screen detection when the disease is asymptomatic to the time when it becomes symptomatic. Looking at the above chart, the length of survival of both patients is the same even though patient A appears to have a longer survival because the cancer was detected earlier, and treatment initiated sooner. Obviously, the credit for a 'longer period of survival' cannot be given to the earlier detection and treatment as in truth both the patients have lived the same total duration. It is not, therefore, true that the patient A has lived longer than patient B. If, however, the patient A does not die at the same endpoint as patient B but lives for longer and dies later at the point 'Y' in the figure, then the earlier detection of the cancer would have been beneficial and the survival longer. To eliminate the lead time bias, therefore, one must verify that the end-point has been moved further because of earlier detection.

Section 9: Treatment of breast cancer

Breast cancers may be located at a single site, *unifocal* or may be *multi-focal or multi-centric.*

- Unifocal (UF) breast cancer is a singular breast carcinoma with a better prognosis.
- Multifocal (MF) – more than one site within the same quadrant separated by benign tissue.
- Multicentric (MC) – cancer in multiple quadrants

(*Source:* Wolters R, Wöckel A, Janni W, Novopashenny I, Ebner F, Kreienberg R, et al. Comparing the outcome between multicentric and multifocal breast cancer: what is the impact on survival, and is there a role for guideline-adherent adjuvant therapy? A retrospective multicenter cohort study of 8,935 patients. Breast Cancer Res Treat 2013; 142:579–590.)

There is ongoing debate as to whether MF/MC is due to the chronology or the biological aggression of the malignancy. Some of these can be occult and the only way of proving this will be following histological examination of a mastectomy specimen with 5-mm slices. When this was done, historic studies showed that a proportion between 1 and 60% of breast cancers can be multifocal/multicentric. The impact of this on the type of management is controversial; however, lobular cancers, large cancers and cancers at a younger age have greater rates of multifocality and multicentricity. This effectively means that the entire breast needs to be treated (with procedures such as mastectomy) even when subject to considering breast conserving surgical procedures.

Treatment options for breast cancer

Surgical management is used to control *loco-regional disease*. While surgery remains critical for many breast cancer cases today, especially for curative intent or staging, the future could see a significant shift towards predominantly medical and non-invasive therapies. Emerging tools like liquid biopsies (blood tests that detect cancer markers) could lead to much earlier diagnoses. This may allow doctors to treat cancers with drugs or other therapies at a stage when surgery is not necessary. Techniques like cryoablation (freezing cancer cells) or high-intensity focussed ultrasound (HIFU) are being explored as alternatives to surgically removing tumours. For the present, however, surgery remains the cornerstone of curative management of breast cancer.

- *Breast conserving surgery* (BCS) in the form of wide local excision (excision of tumour with a rim of normal tissue) or therapeutic mammoplasty (excision of tumour with mobilisation of tissue/flaps/nipple, in the case of large tumours, where the defect is likely to be >20%)
- *Breast resecting surgery* – total mastectomy

Primary treatment for breast cancer is achieved by BCS with radiotherapy or with mastectomy.

Breast reconstruction needs to be considered, where necessary:

- Partial reconstruction (following BCS) is performed commonly using chest wall perforator-based flaps.

- Reconstruction following mastectomy can be performed using silicone implant or tissue flap (i.e. *L*atissimus *D*orsi flap or free flap, such as *D*eep *I*nferior *E*pigastric *A*rtery *P*erforator flap).
- Reduction mammoplasty of the contralateral breast may need consideration.

Lymph nodal clearance is carried out based on the nodal status as assessed where possible by sentinel node biopsy.

Adjuvant therapy or additional therapy

This is the term used to treat or inhibit micro-metastasis after surgery has been undertaken. This takes the form of:

- Radiotherapy (which now can also be delivered during surgery in selected cases, called '*I*ntra-*O*perative *R*adiation *T*herapy')
- Chemotherapy
- Hormonal therapy
- Monoclonal antibody therapy, or
- Various combinations of these

Taking into consideration the prognostic implications, the treatment plan can be made available for individual patients. In general, terms hormonal receptor status, tumour size and nodal status are all independent prognostic predictors.

Neoadjuvant therapy

This type of therapy is the treatment that is given before surgery to decrease the size of cancer and thus enabling local control with surgery.

Standard work-up prior to definitive treatment applies to all.

a. Confirm diagnosis of malignancy with cytology.
b. Confirm grade of malignancy.
c. Confirm nodal status.
d. Confirm hormonal status.

Examples:

1. Management of a post-menopausal 70 years old lady with a screen detected T1NOMO breast cancer.

   Majority of screen detected tumours are small and benefit from breast conserving surgery and radiotherapy, with or without hormonal therapy based on the hormonal status.

2. A 30-year-old pregnant woman with a rapidly increasing breast lump (discussion can focus on inflammatory breast cancer)

   These are aggressive tumours. They are normally ER negative and show evidence of rapid growth. Most of them are advanced at presentation with positive nodes. They tend to occur in the younger age group. They can be mistaken for mastitis as the breast may be inflamed, warm and tender to touch. They occur in young women with dense breast tissue and may elude mammographic detection. Imaging will include ultrasound of breast and nodes, mammogram, CT staging or PET CT.

The treatment options here are:

- Neoadjuvant therapy – chemotherapy
- Targeted therapy as with Herceptin, if appropriate
- Mastectomy with nodal clearance
- Postoperative radiotherapy and possibly delayed reconstruction when appropriate.

3. A 65-year-old man with a palpable lump in the left breast.

   Standard work-up prior to definitive treatment applies to all.

   - Confirm diagnosis of malignancy with cytology.
   - Confirm grade of malignancy.
   - Confirm nodal status.

   Most will be treatable with mastectomy and or nodal clearance; some may need radiotherapy.

4. Management of a 45-year-old lady presenting with a large palpable breast lump of 3 months duration

   - Work-up as discussed.
   - Assessment of hormonal status is important.
   - Triple negative cancers need a different pathway of care.
   - Consider reconstructive mammoplasty.

5. Pre-menopausal lady with a new lump in her left axilla

   The options here are:

   - Clinical and radiological examination of the breasts. MRI may need consideration if no lumps are detected on clinical and mammographic examination.
   - Followed by cytological examination if a lump is detected
   - Ultrasound examination of the axillary lump with FNAC
   - Rest of the management depends on the findings.
   - If a breast primary is not located, an axillary biopsy may be needed as on rare occasions lymphoma can present with a solitary lump.

Prognosis

Assessment of prognosis can be made in different ways.

PREDICT (https://breast.predict.cam/) is often used as a prognostication tool for early IBC.

Example: A 64-year-old post-menopausal woman, diagnosed with symptomatic breast cancer, has undergone surgery.

The final results are as follows: 26 mm, grade 2 invasive, ductal carcinoma NST, ER positive, *HER2* negative, *Ki67* unknown, and two axillary nodes showed macro-metastasis.

Results of the Predict Breast tool, as summarised below (**Figure 5**), show how different treatments would be expected to improve survival rates.

Overall survival
This chart shows the percentage of women surviving 10 years after surgery

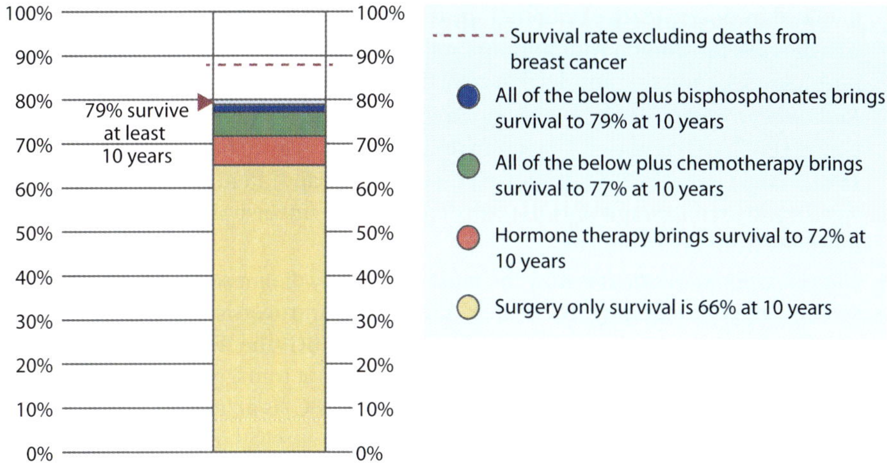

In summary:

- 66 out of 100 women treated with surgery only, are alive at least 10 years from surgery
- 72 out of 100 women treated with hormone therapy are alive (an extra 7)
- 77 out of 100 women treated with hormone therapy, and chemotherapy are alive (an extra 12)
- 79 out of 100 women treated with hormone therapy, chemotherapy, and bisphosphonates are alive (an extra 14)

Of the women who would not survive, 12 would die due to causes not related to breast cancer

Figure 5 The 'Predict Breast' tool.

Section 10: Appendix – interesting papers

1. *National surgical adjuvant breast and bowel project, NSABP B04 trial:* This study started in 1971. 25-year follow-up of a randomised trial comparing radical mastectomy, total mastectomy, and total mastectomy followed by irradiation. Total mastectomy with radiotherapy is not inferior to Halsted radical mastectomy. It also showed that there was no benefit from post mastectomy radiotherapy in node negative breast cancer. Furthermore, the study showed that leaving behind occult positive axillary nodes did not affect rates of distant metastasis or breast cancer related deaths.

   A total of 1,079 women with clinically negative axillary nodes underwent radical mastectomy, total mastectomy without axillary dissection but with postoperative irradiation, or total mastectomy plus axillary dissection only if their nodes became positive. A total of 586 women with clinically positive axillary nodes either underwent radical mastectomy or underwent total mastectomy without axillary dissection but with postoperative irradiation. Kaplan–Meier and cumulative-incidence estimate of outcome were obtained. Results: No significant differences were observed among the three groups of women with negative nodes or between the two groups of women with positive nodes with respect to disease-free survival, relapse-free survival, distant-disease-free survival, or overall survival.

2. *NSABP B-06: 20- year follow-up of a randomised trial comparing total mastectomy, lumpectomy and lumpectomy plus irradiation for IBC.*

   This trial, of 2,163 patients between 1976 and 1984, showed that even a lumpectomy followed by postoperative radiotherapy was an adequate treatment for IBC. This was the case for women with tumours < 4 cm, stages 1 and 2. Lumpectomy with postoperative radiotherapy decreased ipsilateral recurrence.
3. *Radiotherapy after breast conserving surgery:* Early Breast Cancer Trialists Collaborative Group (EBCTCG) reported a meta-analysis of 17 RCTs in 10,801 women from 1976 to 1999, in the Lancet in 2011. It showed that radiotherapy after breast conserving surgery significantly reduced not only the risk of recurrence but also showed a reduction in mortality from breast cancer.
4. *Duct carcinoma in situ:* It is now the most commonly diagnosed abnormality on screening mammography. There are a number of controversies regarding the treatment of DCIS. It is staged as Stage 0 breast cancer or pre-IBC. The IBC transgresses the basement membrane. In DCIS, the cancer cells do not transgress the basement membrane. Progression to invasive breast cancer (IBC) is at least 13–50% over a range of 10 or more years after initial diagnosis. The survival regardless of the mode of treatment provided seems to be excellent. Under these circumstances and because of natural variation in progression, under treatment or over treatment is difficult to judge. DCIS is graded, like IBC into, low, medium and high-grade tumours. The high-grade tumours are more likely to progress to IBC. The modalities of recommended treatment of DCIS are:
   - *Breast conserving surgery* – wide local excision with a clearance of at least 2 mm
   - Followed by *radiotherapy* to the whole breast
   - In *ER + patients,* tamoxifen or aromatase inhibitor may decrease the recurrence in the ipsilateral breast.
5. *Relevance of breast cancer hormone receptors and other factors to the efficacy of adjuvant tamoxifen:* Patient-level meta-analysis of randomised trials. Lancet 2011. *Early Breast Cancer Trialists' Collaborative Group (EBCTCG):* This is a meta-analysis of 21,457 patients of which 10,645 patients were ER positive. It showed that there was a 15-year reduction in death and recurrence from 5 years of treatment with tamoxifen in ER + patients even then the ER was only feebly positive.
6. *Aromatase inhibitors versus tamoxifen in early breast cancer:* Patient-level meta-analysis of the randomised trials. *Early Breast Cancer Trialists' Collaborative Group (EBCTCG):* This study was presented in Lancet in 2015. It was a meta-analysis of 31,920 post-menopausal ER positive early breast cancer patients. It analysed 5 years of tamoxifen versus 5 years of aromatase inhibitors, 5 years of aromatase versus tamoxifen followed by aromatase and aromatase followed by tamoxifen versus tamoxifen alone. It found that 5 years aromatase inhibitor reduces the risk of death from breast cancer at 10 years by 15% compared to 5 years of treatment with tamoxifen.
7. *Adjuvant bisphosphonates reduce the rate of breast cancer recurrence in the bone and improve breast cancer survival,* but there is definite benefit only in women who were postmenopausal when treatment began. Early Breast Cancer Trialists' Collaborative Group (EBCTCG): Taking all women together, regardless of menopausal status, this collaborative meta-analysis of individual patient data from 18,766 women randomised in trials of adjuvant bisphosphonates found a highly significant reduction only in bone

recurrence, and not in other breast cancer outcomes. Subgroup analyses suggested benefit just in postmenopausal women, among whom there were highly significant reductions not only in bone recurrence but also in any distant recurrence (bone or other), breast cancer mortality, and overall mortality.

9. Much more reliable comparisons of different bisphosphonate regimens will emerge from ongoing trials that compare them directly. The SWOG0307 trial (NCT00127205) comparing *clodronate versus zoledronic acid versus ibandronate* in 5,400 patients has completed recruitment and addresses the choice of agent; the SUCCESS trial (NCT02181101) comparing 5 years versus 2 years of zoledronic acid in 3,800 patients has also completed recruitment and addresses duration.

William Halstead – American surgeon (1852–1922)

Halstead was an American surgeon credited with establishing the surgical residency programme in Johns Hopkins Hospital, Baltimore, USA, based on his training in Europe under great surgeons such as Bassini, Kocher, etc.

He learnt techniques of mastectomy and took it to higher levels in the belief of '*eradicating*' the cancer by its 'roots'. Hence, the term '*radical*' *mastectomy* – a mutilating operation that disfigured women based on the then prevailing concept of '*cut more-cure more*'.

He kept a meticulous record of his operations and results. The realisation must have dawned on him that he could not cure more by cutting more, as patients he had expected to cure died of the disease due to metastasis.

He also learnt, in Europe, that cocaine drops in the eye had anaesthetic properties and in the process of trying it out himself became addicted to cocaine!

He married his theatre sister and as she had contact dermatitis to the chemicals used for sterilising, he contacted the 'Good Year' company and had special rubber gloves made for her. Although not initially for sterility purpose, this became established as good surgical practice throughout the world.

Chapter 4

Upper gastrointestinal malignancies

Ilias Marios Oikonomou, Marena Gray, Vlasios Gourgiotis, Stavros Gourgiotis, Srinivasan Ravi

Introduction

Upper gastrointestinal (UGI) malignancies encompass cancers arising in the oesophagus, stomach, and duodenum, each with distinct anatomical locations, biological behaviours, and clinical presentations.

Section 1: Anatomy of the upper gastrointestinal tract (Figures 1 and 2)

The UGI tract begins at the oesophagus, a muscular tube approximately 25–30 cm long, extending from the pharynx to the stomach. The oesophagus passes through the thoracic

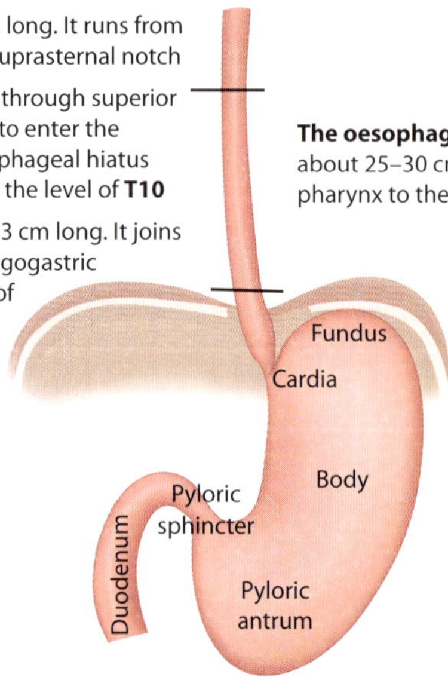

Figure 1 Anatomy of the upper gastrointestinal tract.

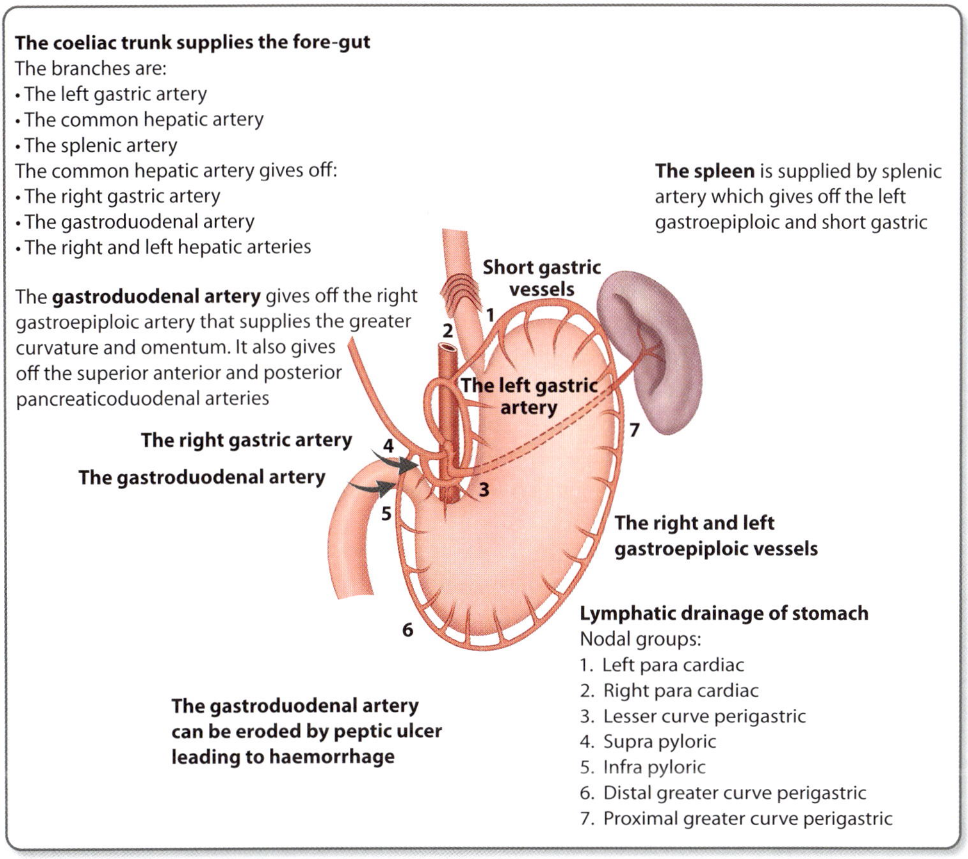

Figure 2 Basic anatomy – blood supply and nodes.

cavity, traversing the diaphragm via the oesophageal hiatus, and terminates at the gastroesophageal junction.

The stomach lies primarily in the left upper quadrant of the abdomen and is divided into anatomical regions: the cardia, fundus, body, and pylorus. The gastric wall consists of four layers: mucosa, submucosa, muscularis propria and serosa, each playing a role in malignancy progression.

The pancreas, a retroperitoneal organ, has three parts: the head (adjacent to the duodenum), body and tail (extending towards the spleen). The pancreatic duct merges with the common bile duct, emptying into the duodenum via the ampulla of Vater.

Section 2: Gastro-oesophageal cancers

The distal gastric cancers have decreased over the years but have stabilised since 2002. There is a link between distal gastric cancers and *Helicobacter pylori (H. pylori)*. As the cohort of the population with *H. pylori* decreased, so did the distal gastric cancers. This is not the case with the cancers in the gastro-oesophageal region. Their proportion and numbers have increased steadily and this may relate to the change in the demographics of the population as well as the increase in *obesity*.

Gastrointestinal reflux disease of over 10 or more years leads to *Barrett's oesophagus.* Gastro-oesophageal reflux disease (GORD) leads to changes in the nature of the mucosa referred to as metaplasia and predisposes to neoplastic change over years. Early detection, treatment and monitoring of this has a role in prevention of the dreaded adenocarcinoma in the lower oesophagus involving the cardia.

Common types of upper gastrointestinal malignancies

1. *Oesophagus:*
   - *Adenocarcinoma* most commonly arises in the lower third, often associated with Barrett's oesophagus.
   - *Squamous cell carcinoma* occurs predominantly in the upper and middle thirds, linked to smoking and alcohol.
2. *Stomach:* The most common type of gastric cancer is adenocarcinoma, which accounts for about 90% of all malignancies. Adenocarcinomas typically arise from the mucosal gland cells. Other types of gastric malignancies include gastrointestinal stromal tumours (GIST), neuroendocrine tumours and lymphomas.
3. *Duodenum:* Duodenal cancer is rare, but it is aggressive. It usually arises from the 3rd or 4th part of the duodenum and it is most commonly *adenocarcinoma.*

The lower oesophagus and stomach, being derivatives of the endoderm, are lined with columnar epithelium. These give rise to adenocarcinoma.

Lymphomas and *MALTomas* (*M*ucosa *A*ssociated *L*ymphoid *T*issue MALT lymphoma) occur in the stomach. This is a type of non-Hodgkins lymphoma associated with B lymphocytes and to *H. pylori* infections.

Upper GI cancers may relate to *familial adenomatous polyposis (FAP), Lynch syndrome and Peutz-Jegers syndrome (GI polyposis).*

Regional variation

1. *Oesophageal cancer:*
   - Increasing prevalence of *adenocarcinoma* in Western countries is attributed to obesity and GORD.
   - *Squamous cell carcinoma* mainly dominates in Asia and Africa, driven by tobacco, alcohol, and dietary carcinogens.
2. *Gastric cancer:*
   - East Asia, particularly Japan and South Korea, report the highest incidence, partly due to *H. pylori* infection and dietary factors.
   - Non-cardia gastric cancer is decreasing globally, while cardia cancer incidence is rising in Western populations.

Section 3: Risk factors and genetic syndromes

The development of UGI malignancies is influenced by a complex interplay of genetic predisposition, environmental factors, and lifestyle behaviours.

Oesophageal cancers:

- Ageing over 70s is predominantly affected.
- Obesity

- Reflux disease
- Barrat's oesophagus
- Smoking
- Alcohol consumption
- Diet poor in vegetables and fruit

Gastric cancers:
- *H. pylori* for mid and distal gastric cancers
- Chronic atrophic gastritis
- Diet, high in salt
- Incidence is 2–3 times higher in male patients
- High-salt diets, smoking, and genetic predispositions

Genetic syndromes associated with UGI malignancies

1. *Lynch syndrome (hereditary nonpolyposis colorectal cancer, HNPCC):*
    - Lynch syndrome, caused by mutations in mismatch repair genes (e.g. *MLH1* and *MSH2*), predisposes individuals to various cancers, including gastric and pancreatic cancer. Gastric cancer in Lynch syndrome often arises from intestinal-type adenocarcinoma.
    - Screening for Lynch syndrome in high-risk families involves genetic testing and endoscopic surveillance.
2. *Familial adenomatous polyposis (FAP):* FAP, caused by mutations in the *APC* gene, is associated with a markedly increased risk of duodenal and gastric adenomas, some of which may progress to adenocarcinoma.

   Surveillance programmes include regular UGI endoscopies to detect and manage premalignant lesions.
3. *BRCA mutations:* Germline mutations in *BRCA1* and *BRCA2,* classically associated with breast and ovarian cancers, also elevate the risk of pancreatic cancer.

   BRCA pathogenic variations in combination with *H. pylori* infection increase the lifetime risk of gastric cancer.
4. *CDH1 mutations:* Mutations in the *CDH1* gene, encoding E-cadherin, predispose carriers to hereditary diffuse gastric cancer (HDGC) and lobular breast cancer.
5. *Peutz-Jeghers syndrome (PJS):* PJS is characterised by mutations in the *STK11* gene, leading to hamartomatous polyps throughout the gastrointestinal tract and an increased risk of pancreatic and gastric cancers.

Environmental and lifestyle risk factors

1. *Helicobacter pylori infection:* Chronic *H. pylori* infection is a well-established risk factor for non-cardia gastric cancer. The bacterium induces chronic inflammation, atrophic gastritis, and intestinal metaplasia, creating a pathway to malignancy.
    - Because of its role in causing gastric cancer in 1994, *H. pylori* was classified as a human carcinogen or cancer-causing agent, by the World Health Organisation's International Agency for Research on Cancer.
    - Risk of gastric cancer was reduced statistically in high-risk individuals when treated with *H. pylori* eradication, ascorbic acid or β-carotene (https://doi.org/10.1093/jnci/92.23.1881).

2. *Dietary factors:*
    - *High salt and nitrate intake:* Diets rich in salted, smoked, or pickled foods are linked to gastric cancer.
    - *Low fruit and vegetable consumption:* Antioxidants and dietary fibre from fruits and vegetables have protective effects against UGI cancers.
3. *Obesity:* Excess adiposity contributes to GORD, a precursor to oesophageal adenocarcinoma.
4. *Tobacco and alcohol use:* Smoking is a major risk factor for oesophageal, gastric, and pancreatic cancers, with dose-dependent effects.

    Chronic alcohol consumption increases the risk of oesophageal squamous cell carcinoma and synergistically exacerbates the effects of smoking.
5. *Gastro-oesophageal reflux disease and Barrett's oesophagus: GORD,* characterised by chronic acid exposure in the lower oesophagus, leads to Barrett's oesophagus, a condition involving metaplastic columnar epithelium replacement of the squamous lining.

Barrett's oesophagus is the precursor lesion for oesophageal adenocarcinoma.

Emerging risk factors

1. *Microbiome alterations:* Dysbiosis, or alterations in the gut microbiota, is increasingly recognised as a contributor to UGI malignancies. Certain bacterial species, such as *Fusobacterium nucleatum,* are associated with tumourigenesis.
2. *Metabolic syndrome:* Components of metabolic syndrome, including insulin resistance and hyperlipidaemia, have been linked to pancreatic cancer development.

Section 4: Barrett's oesophagus and dysplasia

Barrett's oesophagus represents a precancerous condition in the development of oesophageal adenocarcinoma. It is characterised by the *replacement of normal squamous epithelium with columnar epithelium* in the distal oesophagus, Barrett's oesophagus arises because of chronic GORD.

Pathophysiology of Barrett's oesophagus

1. *Role of chronic GORD:* Repeated exposure to gastric acid and bile leads to epithelial injury and subsequent metaplastic transformation of squamous cells into columnar cells resembling *intestinal epithelium.*
2. *Molecular pathogenesis:*
    - Genetic alterations such as *TP53* mutations and loss of heterozygosity are observed early in the progression from Barrett's oesophagus to oesophageal adenocarcinoma.
    - Overexpression of cyclooxygenase-2 (COX-2) and activation of the Wnt/β-catenin pathway further drive dysplasia and malignancy.

Risk factors for Barrett's oesophagus

1. *GORD symptoms:* Chronic heartburn and acid regurgitation are the primary risk factors.
2. *Obesity and central adiposity:* Excess visceral fat increases intra-abdominal pressure, exacerbating GORD.

3. *Male sex and age:* Barrett's oesophagus is more prevalent in men and individuals over 50 years.
4. *Smoking:* Smoking is a modifiable risk factor that doubles the risk of Barrett's oesophagus.

Diagnosis and surveillance

1. *Endoscopic diagnosis:*
    - Barrett's oesophagus is diagnosed via endoscopy, with biopsies confirming the presence of specialised intestinal metaplasia.
    - The *Prague classification system* can be used to measure the extent of Barrett's oesophagus by circumferential and maximal length (C and M criteria). For example, M4C3 will mean involvement of 4 cm length and 3 cm of circumference.
2. *Surveillance guidelines:*
    - Regular endoscopic surveillance is recommended for patients with confirmed Barrett's oesophagus to detect dysplasia or early cancer.
    - Frequency of surveillance depends on the presence and grade of dysplasia. Local or national guidelines should be sought and followed to establish appropriate surveillance periods.

Dysplasia in Barrett's oesophagus

1. *Classification of dysplasia:* Dysplasia is categorised as *low-grade or high-grade* based on histopathological criteria. High-grade dysplasia has a significant risk of progression to adenocarcinoma.
2. *Progression to oesophageal adenocarcinoma:* Patients with Barrett's oesophagus have a 0.1–0.3% annual risk of developing oesophageal adenocarcinoma. This risk increases substantially with high-grade dysplasia.

Management strategies

1. *Endoscopic therapy:*
    - *Endoscopic mucosal resection (EMR):* Effective for removing visible lesions and obtaining larger tissue samples for histology.
    - *Radiofrequency ablation (RFA):* Used to eradicate residual Barrett's epithelium following EMR or in patients with dysplasia.
2. *Pharmacological therapy: Proton pump inhibitors (PPIs) are the cornerstone of medical management,* reducing acid exposure and promoting healing.
3. *Surgical intervention:* Oesophagectomy remains an option for patients with high-grade dysplasia or early-stage adenocarcinoma not amenable to endoscopic therapy.

Preventive strategies

1. *Lifestyle modifications:* Weight loss, dietary changes, and smoking cessation are essential for reducing GORD severity and Barrett's progression.
2. *Chemoprevention:* Studies suggest potential benefits of aspirin and PPIs in reducing progression to dysplasia.

Section 5: Clinical presentations in upper gastrointestinal malignancies

Oesophageal cancer

Clinical presentation can include any combination of the following and symptoms:

- *Dysphagia:* Progressive dysphagia typically starts with solids and progresses to liquids, reflecting lumen obstruction. Associated with weight loss due to reduced oral intake.
- *Weight loss:* Unexplained loss of 10% of body weight in 3–6 months
- *Odynophagia:* Painful swallowing, often indicating ulceration or invasion of adjacent structures.
- *Retrosternal pain:* Suggests advanced disease with mediastinal involvement or nerve invasion.
- *Hoarseness:* Results from recurrent laryngeal nerve involvement, often signifying advanced disease.
- *Haematemesis and melaena:* Occur due to tumour ulceration and bleeding.

Gastric cancer

In gastric cancer, the clinical picture may have a more diverse presentation. Some of the most common symptoms are:

- *Epigastric pain:* A common presenting symptom, often non-specific and mistaken for peptic ulcer disease.
- *Early satiety:* Indicates reduced stomach capacity due to tumour infiltration or obstruction.
- *Nausea and vomiting:* Vomiting may occur with proximal gastric or gastro-oesophageal junction tumours causing obstruction.
- *Unintentional weight loss:* Reflects cancer cachexia, anorexia, or obstruction-induced malnutrition.
- *Haematemesis and anaemia:* Occult bleeding or overt haematemesis may result from ulcerated tumours.
- *Epigastric mass:* While a rarer symptom, a palpable epigastric mass should always alert the clinician. When accompanied with weight loss or haematemesis, the patient should be referred for further assessment.

Duodenal cancer

- *Obstructive symptoms:*
  - *Biliary obstruction:* Presents with jaundice, dark urine, and pale stools due to ampullary involvement.
  - *Duodenal obstruction:* Causes postprandial vomiting, epigastric distension, and pain.
- *Constitutional symptoms:* Non-specific symptoms such as fatigue and weight loss are common.

Advanced disease presentations

UGI cancers frequently present late, often with metastatic symptoms:

- Liver metastases cause hepatomegaly, jaundice, and ascites.

- Peritoneal carcinomatosis manifests as ascites and abdominal discomfort.
- Bone metastases lead to bone pain and pathological fractures.
- Pulmonary metastases result in dyspnoea, cough, and haemoptysis.

Paraneoplastic syndromes

Rarely, UGI malignancies may present with paraneoplastic syndromes:

- *Acanthosis nigricans:* Associated with gastric cancer, characterised by hyperpigmented, velvety plaques in skin folds. Its appearance is considered *a poor prognostic factor.*
- *Hypercoagulability:* Trousseau's syndrome (migratory thrombophlebitis) is linked to advanced malignancy.

Referral guidance (NICE 2015)

The 2-week wait pathway

For UGI malignancies, referral is warranted if patients present with the following:

1. *Dysphagia:* Any new or progressive difficulty in swallowing should prompt immediate referral.
2. *Over-55 years with unexplained weight loss:* Especially if associated with upper abdominal pain, reflux, or dyspepsia, plus one of the following:
    a. *Epigastric mass:* A palpable mass in the upper abdomen is highly suggestive of advanced disease.
    b. *Persistent dyspepsia:* Persistent or worsening symptoms, particularly in individuals with additional risk factors.
    c. *Reflux symptoms:* Any reflux symptomatology not responding well to PPI.
    d. *Upper abdominal pain:* Subacute upper abdominal pain that has been established for a short period of time and does not have the characteristics of an acute condition.

Additional criteria include persistent vomiting, jaundice, or significant family history of gastrointestinal malignancies.

Non-urgent referral

Patients with less severe symptoms may still warrant non-urgent referral if conservative management fails or symptoms persist. For example:

- Chronic GORD symptoms not responding to PPIs
- Ongoing dyspepsia with no identifiable benign cause
- Upper abdominal pain with low haemoglobin levels
- *Iron deficiency anaemia:* A possible indicator of chronic gastrointestinal blood loss.

It is always important to apply the latest guideline for urgent and non-urgent referrals, as they are often renewed, when there is new knowledge available.

Section 6: Diagnosis and staging of upper gastrointestinal malignancies

The accurate diagnosis and staging of the UGI malignancies are fundamental to determining the appropriate treatment and predicting patient outcomes. These processes involve a combination of:

- Clinical assessment
- Laboratory investigations
- Imaging studies
- Advanced endoscopic techniques

Clinical assessment and presentation

The clinical manifestations of UGI cancers are often subtle in their early stages, contributing to *delayed diagnosis*. Patients may present with symptoms such as dysphagia, epigastric pain, unintentional weight loss, or fatigue. Alarm symptoms, including haematemesis, melaena, or persistent vomiting, may indicate advanced disease. A thorough history and physical examination are crucial in identifying risk factors such as *H. pylori* infection, smoking, or a family history of malignancy.

Laboratory investigations

Initial diagnostic work-up often includes basic laboratory tests to evaluate overall health and organ function.

- *Full blood count (FBC):* Anaemia, often microcytic, may suggest chronic blood loss from a malignancy.
- *Liver function tests (LFTs):* Abnormalities may indicate liver metastases, particularly elevated alkaline phosphatase or transaminases.
- *Tumour markers:* These are of limited value in diagnosis but may have a value in monitoring response to treatment.
  - *Carcinoembryonic antigen (CEA):* Elevated in gastric and pancreatic cancers. *CA 19-9:* Frequently elevated in pancreatic and biliary cancers.
  - *Alpha-fetoprotein (AFP):* Associated with hepatocellular carcinoma but may be seen in rare gastric tumours.

Imaging modalities

Imaging plays a major role in detecting primary tumours, evaluating local invasion, and identifying distant metastases. The choice of modality depends on the clinical scenario and suspected site of malignancy.

- *Ultrasound:* Often the initial imaging modality for suspected pancreatic or liver masses, offering a non-invasive and cost-effective assessment. Nevertheless, it is significantly user dependent and has limited value in the imaging of gastric and oesophageal masses.
- *Computed tomography (CT):* CT with contrast enhancement is the key to staging gastric, oesophageal, and pancreatic cancers. It provides detailed information on tumour size, lymph node involvement, and distant spread.

- *Magnetic resonance imaging (MRI):* Particularly useful for hepatic lesions, biliary tract assessment, and detecting peritoneal carcinomatosis.
- *Positron emission tomography (PET)-CT:* Enhances the detection of metastatic disease and helps to differentiate between malignant and benign lesions.

Histopathological diagnosis

Definitive diagnosis relies on histological confirmation obtained via biopsy. Sampled tissue is histopathologically assessed for malignancy, and grading of the tumour based on cellular differentiation. Immunohistochemistry may be employed to identify specific markers that aid in diagnosis or guide targeted therapies, such as *HER2* in gastric cancer or *PD-L1* in oesophageal cancer.

Staging systems

Accurate staging is crucial for guiding treatment and estimating prognosis. The *T*umour, *N*ode, and *M*etastasis (TNM) classification, established by the American Joint Committee on Cancer (AJCC), is universally employed and is the standard framework for staging. The TNM staging for gastric and oesophageal (**Figure 3**) is similar with minor discrepancies per type.

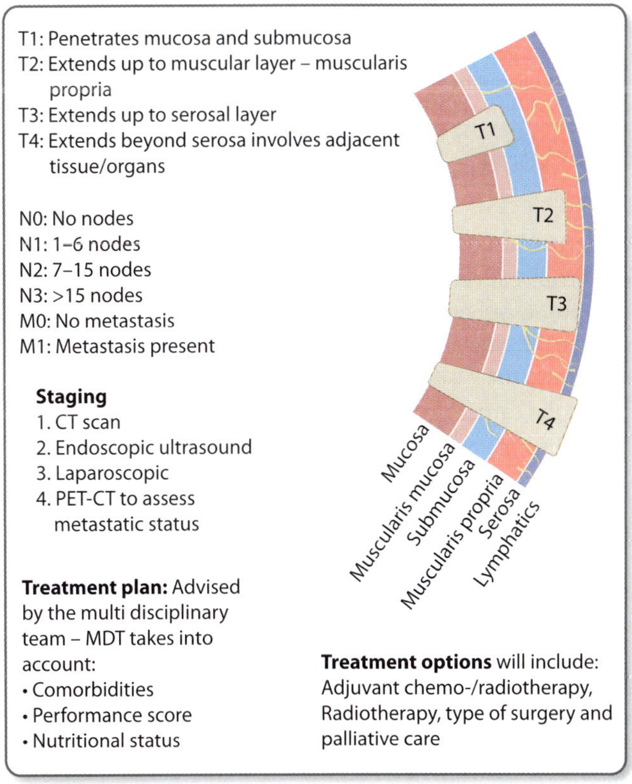

Figure 3 The TNM staging for gastric and oesophageal cancer.

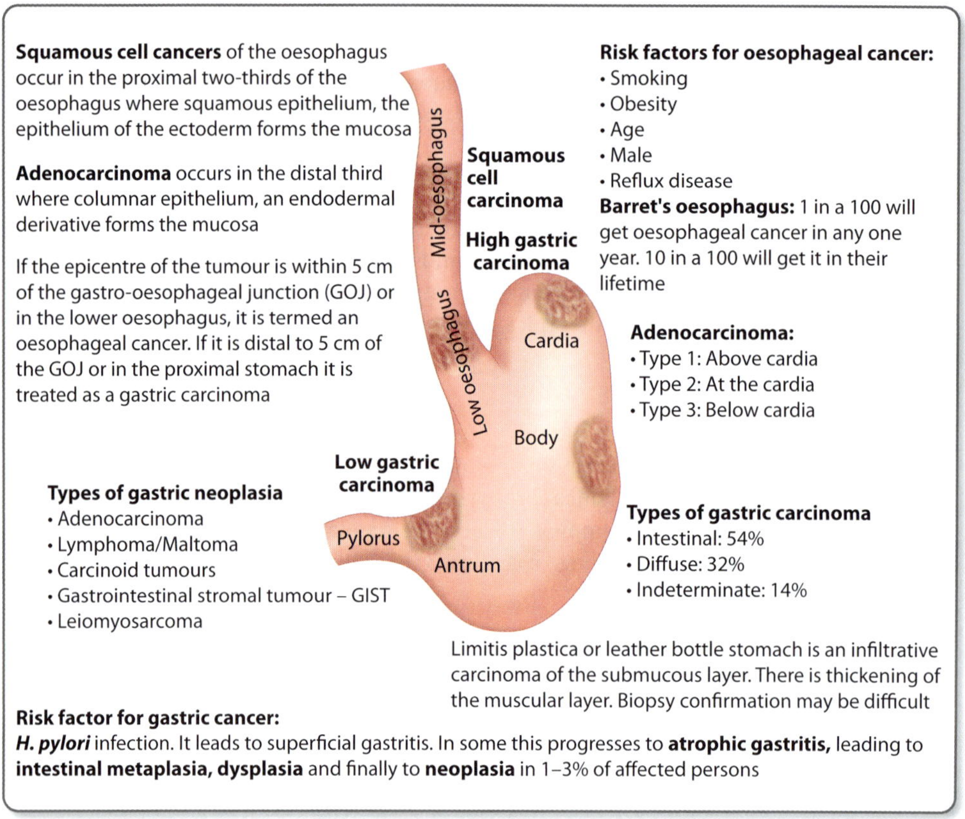

Figure 4 Key features of oesophago-gastric cancer.

Categories of gastro-oesophageal cancers (Figure 4)

The treatment of gastric and oesophageal cancers being different, it is important to categorise the tumours at the gastro-oesophageal junction into either gastric or oesophageal in origin. To address this, the cancers in this area are categorised into:

- Type 1 adenocarcinoma located above the cardia
- Type 2 adenocarcinoma located at the cardia
- Type 3 adenocarcinoma located below the cardia

Section 7: Investigations and assessment

Once the diagnosis is suspected histological confirmation will be needed followed by staging investigations.

Endoscopic techniques

Endoscopy is indispensable for diagnosing and staging UGI malignancies, offering both visualisation and tissue sampling.

- *Oesophagogastroduodenoscopy (OGD):* Essential for identifying and taking biopsies of oesophageal and gastric lesions. High-definition imaging and chromoendoscopy enhance the detection of subtle abnormalities.

- *Endoscopic ultrasound* particularly to help to delineate the level of involvement of the wall of the oesophagus in early tumours and clearly define the 'T' stage. It will also assist in the cytological sampling of adjacent nodes for presence of involvement. Early tumours when identified may be managed with *EMR – endomucosal resection.*

Imaging techniques and laparoscopy

- *CT scan* with contrast enhancement is crucial for site, size, and extent of spread.
- *Ultrasound scan* is useful for staging liver metastases.
- *Magnetic resonance imaging (MRI):* Particularly useful for hepatic lesions, biliary tract assessment, and detecting peritoneal carcinomatosis.
- *Positron emission tomography (PET-CT)* scan enables detection of metastasis that is suspected on CT scan. It can differentiate between malignant and benign lesions.
- *Laparoscopic assessment* for gastric tumours will assist in planning management and aid in the collection of peritoneal samples for cytology; the cytology, if positive, may mean offering only palliative rather than radical treatment; the studies are not yet clear on the benefits of cytological assessment.

The assessment must also take into consideration other factors that might alter the type of treatment offered.

Performance score plays a major role in the decision-making process as the treatment is often very challenging and may not be suitable for all. As always, the feasibility of a treatment is not an indication to provide it. Holistic attitude, viewing the patient's overall status of health, is necessary.

Nutritional status needs careful assessment and preparation if radical treatment is on offer.

When radical treatment is not offered, then palliative care or symptom relief must be put into place.

Section 8: Management of gastric cancer

TNM staging as seen earlier remains the mainstay of management allowing for the appropriate management depending on the factors highlighted above. In western countries, these cancers are treated in specialist units dedicated to the treatment of UGI cancers. Decisions in the UK are collectively taken in multidisciplinary units that involve oncologists and radiologists in deciding an agreed optimal treatment plan for every individual patient. This is understandably not universal due to varying patterns of health care across the globe.

Treatment

Effective management aims to eradicate the tumour, control symptoms, and improve survival while maintaining quality of life. Treatment modalities include surgery, systemic therapies, and radiation, often in combination.

- *Surgical resection* and reconstruction – subtotal or total gastrectomy offers the possibility of a curative treatment provided the malignancy is confined to the primary source.
- *Peri-operative chemotherapy* as recommended by the oncologists in the multidisciplinary team meeting. This could be pre-operative (neoadjuvant) or

postoperative (adjuvant). Common regimens include fluorouracil, leucovorin, oxaliplatin, and docetaxel (FLOT) or cisplatin-based combinations.
- *Postoperative chemoradiotherapy*
- *Postoperative chemotherapy*
- *Palliative care* is aimed at symptom control and quality of life in advanced-stage disease.
  - *Endoscopic stenting:* Provides relief for obstructive symptoms in oesophageal or gastric cancers.
  - *Pain management:* Employs multimodal approaches, including opioids and nerve blocks.
  - *Nutritional support:* Enteral feeding through gastrostomy or jejunostomy may be necessary.

At all times the aim here is to improve the quality of residual life.

Minimally invasive surgery

Minimally invasive surgery (MIS), encompassing laparoscopic and robotic-assisted procedures, has become increasingly prevalent in the management of UGI malignancies. These techniques offer distinct benefits, including reduced postoperative pain, shorter hospital stays, and faster recovery times, while achieving oncological outcomes comparable to traditional approaches.
- *Laparoscopic surgery:* This approach is widely utilised for gastric and oesophageal cancers. Studies have shown that laparoscopic gastrectomy provides equivalent survival rates to open surgery for early-stage gastric cancer, with significantly reduced morbidity.
- *Robotic-assisted surgery:* Offers improved precision and visualisation. Robotic surgery is particularly advantageous in complex anatomical areas such as the mediastinum and gastroesophageal junction. Early results suggest that robotic oesophagectomy may reduce complications like anastomotic leakage compared to open techniques.

Section 9: Screening and referral in upper gastrointestinal malignancies

Screening and timely referral are critical components in improving outcomes for upper gastrointestinal (UGI) malignancies, where early detection significantly increases the likelihood of curative treatment.

The rationale for screening

Screening for UGI malignancies aims to identify high-risk individuals before symptoms develop, enabling intervention at an earlier, more treatable stage. UGI cancers often present late due to vague or non-specific symptoms, contributing to poor prognosis. For example:
- *Oesophageal cancer:* Early-stage tumours are often asymptomatic with dysphagia occurring only once significant narrowing of the lumen has occurred.
- *Gastric cancer:* Early symptoms such as dyspepsia or epigastric discomfort are common in benign conditions, delaying diagnosis.

Screening is particularly valuable in populations with a high prevalence of risk factors, such as *H. pylori* infection, Barrett's oesophagus, or familial cancer syndromes.

Current UK screening programmes

Despite its potential, the UK has no national population-wide screening programme for UGI cancers. Instead, targeted screening approaches focus on individuals at higher risk based on clinical and demographic criteria.

Barrett's oesophagus

Barrett's oesophagus is a precancerous condition characterised by metaplastic changes in the oesophageal epithelium, often secondary to chronic GORD. Patients with Barrett's oesophagus are at increased risk of developing oesophageal adenocarcinoma.

- *Surveillance protocols:* Patients with Barrett's oesophagus undergo regular endoscopic surveillance, typically every 2–5 years, depending on dysplasia grade. The European Society of Gastrointestinal Endoscopy suggests an OGD every 5 years for Barrett's oesophagus extending 1–3 cm, and every 3 years for Barrett's extending 3–10 cm. Individualised plans should be made for larger changes. Biopsies are performed using the Seattle protocol, targeting four-quadrant samples every 1–2 cm of the Barrett's segment.

Helicobacter pylori and gastric cancer

The association between *H. pylori* infection and gastric cancer is well-established. In regions with high *H. pylori* prevalence, eradication strategies are a cornerstone of gastric cancer prevention.

- *Targeted screening:* Testing and eradication are recommended for patients with peptic ulcer disease, dyspepsia, or a family history of gastric cancer.

Familial syndromes

Familial cancer syndromes, such as Lynch syndrome or hereditary diffuse gastric cancer, warrant focussed screening.

- *Gastroscopy:* High-risk individuals may undergo regular endoscopy with biopsy to detect early malignancy.
- *Genetic testing:* Carriers of pathogenic mutations in genes such as *CDH1* (for diffuse gastric cancer) are often offered prophylactic gastrectomy.

Oesophagogastroduodenoscopy

Oesophagogastroduodenoscopy remains the gold standard for evaluating patients with alarm symptoms or high-risk features. There are several 'Biopsy Protocols' available; in all of them, multiple biopsies are taken from suspicious lesions, ulcer margins, or Barrett's oesophagus segments.

Screening beyond endoscopy

Emerging technologies are being explored for non-invasive screening:

- *Cytosponge:* A minimally invasive device for collecting oesophageal cells is used in Barrett's oesophagus detection. It has shown promise in large-scale studies.

- *Liquid biopsy:* Analysing circulating tumour DNA (ctDNA) or other biomarkers in the blood for early cancer detection.

Challenges and limitations

Access and equity

Access to endoscopy services varies with significant pressure on NHS resources. Long waiting times may delay diagnosis, particularly in low-risk patients.

Symptom overlap

Many alarm symptoms of UGI malignancies overlap with benign conditions, such as peptic ulcer disease or functional dyspepsia, leading to both over- and under-referral.

Future directions

Risk stratification

Enhanced risk stratification tools could refine referral pathways, prioritising high-risk patients. For example, a combination of clinical risk factors with genetic and molecular biomarkers or artificial intelligence (AI) algorithms analysing patient's records and imaging.

Expansion of non-invasive screening

Non-invasive methods, such as 'Cytosponge' and liquid biopsies, may reduce reliance on endoscopy, improving screening coverage and efficiency.

Section 10: Prognosis and survivorship in upper gastrointestinal malignancies

Prognosis in UGI malignancies varies widely depending on tumour type, stage, and response to treatment. Advances in care have improved survival rates for some patients, but challenges remain in addressing recurrence and long-term complications.

Determinants of prognosis

Tumour stage at diagnosis

- *Localised disease:* Early-stage tumours (e.g. Stage I) have the best outcomes.
- *Advanced disease:* Poor prognosis in metastatic or unresectable cases.

Tumour biology

- *Histological subtype:* Diffuse gastric cancer (Lauren classification) often has a worse prognosis compared to the intestinal type.
- *Molecular markers: HER2* positivity in gastric cancer indicates better response to trastuzumab.

Treatment response

- *Surgical margins:* Negative margins improve survival.
- *Chemotherapy sensitivity:* Tumours responsive to systemic therapies show better outcomes.

Table 1 The 5-year survival rates.	
Extent of involvement	**5-year survival**
Localised: Limited to stomach alone	75%
Regional: Limited to nodes	35%
Distant: Metastatic	7%
All SEER stages combined	36%

Survival in gastric cancer

This depends on many factors including the prior health of the patient and the involvement of lymph nodes.

According to the National Cancer Institute's SEER database (Surveillance, Epidemiology and End Results) 2023 update, the 5-year survival (**Table 1**) is dependent on the stage of the disease when it is first diagnosed.

Long-term survivorship challenges

Recurrence

- *Pattern of recurrence:*
  - Locoregional recurrence in gastric cancer
  - Distant metastases in oesophageal cancer
- *Monitoring:* Regular imaging and endoscopic surveillance.

Functional impairments

- *Post-surgical issues:*
  - Dumping syndrome and nutritional deficiencies after gastrectomy
  - Reduced oesophageal motility post-oesophagectomy
- *Management:* Diet modification, enzyme supplements, and physiotherapy.

Psychosocial impact

- *Emotional well-being:* Survivors may experience depression, anxiety, and post-traumatic stress.
- *Support systems:* Psycho-oncology services and survivor networks play critical roles.

Role of palliative care

- *End-of-life care:* Focusses on comfort and dignity.
- *Symptom management:* Pain, nausea, and dyspnoea relief improve quality of life.

Section 11: Radiotherapy, chemotherapy and targeted therapy for upper gastrointestinal malignancies

Systemic therapies, including chemotherapy and targeted treatments, are integral to the multidisciplinary management of UGI cancers.

Radiotherapy in UGI cancers may be used in the following ways:

- Attempt shrinking the malignancy prior to an operation as neoadjuvant therapy.
- Administered alone or in parallel with chemotherapy, in a chemoradiation protocol.
- Administered postoperatively, as adjuvant therapy, attempting to eradicate any remaining cancer cells.
- Offered as palliative care to ease symptomatology such as pain, bleeding or trouble in swallowing

External beam radiation therapy (EBRT) is the most common type of radiotherapy offered in UGI malignancies. In oesophageal cancer, an *internal radiation therapy model* could be used with the support of an endoscope; this is mainly used for palliative purposes.

Chemotherapy in upper gastrointestinal cancers

Neoadjuvant chemotherapy

Administering chemotherapy prior to surgery aims to downstage tumours, improves resectability, and addresses micrometastatic disease.

Adjuvant chemotherapy

Postoperative chemotherapy aims to eradicate residual microscopic disease, reducing recurrence risk.

Palliative chemotherapy

For metastatic or unresectable cancers, chemotherapy improves symptom control and extends survival.

Targeted therapies

Targeted therapies revolutionise treatment by exploiting specific molecular aberrations within tumour cells.

HER2-targeted therapy

HER2 overexpression occurs in ~20% of gastric and gastroesophageal junction cancers. *Trastuzumab,* a monoclonal antibody, improves survival in *HER2*-positive advanced gastric cancer when combined with chemotherapy.

Vascular endothelial growth factor inhibitors

Targeting angiogenesis is critical in advanced disease management. *Ramucirumab,* a VEGFR-2 antagonist, is used alone or with paclitaxel in refractory gastric cancer.

Section 12: Complications of upper gastrointestinal malignancies and their management

Early recognition of complications and effective management are essential in mitigating morbidity and prolonging survival.
Complications may be:

- Local due to tumour growth and invasion
- Metastatic

Local complications

1. *Dysphagia and obstruction* where luminal narrowing impedes food and liquid passage. This is managed by:
   - *Endoscopic stenting:* Metallic or plastic stents provide rapid relief.
   - *Dilatation:* Balloon or bougie dilators are used, though recurrence rates are high.
   - *Bypass surgery:* In cases where tumours are unresectable, gastrojejunostomy or oesophageal bypass may restore patency.
2. *Haemorrhage* occurs due to erosion of tumour into major vessels, leading to life-threatening bleeding. This is managed by:
   - *Endoscopic intervention:* Techniques like argon plasma coagulation (APC) or clipping.
   - *Radiotherapy:* Palliative radiotherapy (styptic) can help to control bleeding in advanced cases.
   - *Surgical intervention:* In cases of uncontrolled bleeding, surgical intervention is often required as a definitive measure. Options include:
     - *Resection:* Removal of the affected segment.
     - *Ligation:* Tying off the bleeding vessel to halt haemorrhage.
     - *Combined approaches:* Surgery may be complemented by endoscopic techniques or radiotherapy to address residual disease and prevent recurrence.
3. *Perforation:* The management options are guided by multiple factors the most important of which is the overall prognosis for any given patient. In most cases, this likely to be palliative.
   - *Conservative management:* Broad-spectrum coverage to treat peritonitis, bowel rest and close monitoring can be utilised in some cases. Escalation to an operative approach may be required.
   - *Emergency surgery:* The approaches described below are more commonly used in colorectal cases; they are of value in a few selected cases, depending upon the overall prognosis; nevertheless, they may be required in UGI or small bowel cases as well. Specific approaches include:
     - *Primary repair:* Direct suturing of the perforated site.
     - *Segmental resection:* Surgical removal of the affected segment of the gastrointestinal tract, which may be accompanied by restoration of continuity, depending on the patient's condition and tumour location.
     - *Diversion procedures:* In very selected cases with creation of a stoma.
4. *Fistula formation* may be managed with:
   - *Endoscopic stents* that seal fistulae and restore luminal integrity.
   - *Surgical bypass:* Indicated in selected patients with preserved function.

Metastatic complications

Liver metastases present with jaundice, hepatomegaly, and right upper quadrant pain: They may be treated with chemotherapy and targeted agents to control tumour burden. Or, with *ablative techniques such as* radiofrequency ablation (RFA), histotripsy with ultrasound, or transarterial chemoembolisation (TACE) for isolated lesions.

Peritoneal carcinomatosis present with ascites, abdominal pain, and bowel obstruction: In selected patients they can be managed by *Paracentesis* for symptomatic relief of ascites.

Hyperthermic intraperitoneal chemotherapy (HIPEC): It can be used in selected patients with limited peritoneal disease.

Bone metastases may present with pain, pathological fractures, and hypercalcaemia. *Bisphosphonates or denosumab can be used to* reduce skeletal-related events.

Palliative radiotherapy: Controls pain and stabilises fractures.

Pulmonary metastases present with dyspnoea, cough, and pleural effusion. *Thoracocentesis may help in symptomatic relief. Chemotherapy may* help to control tumour progression.

In the palliative management of metastatic upper GI cancer, and perhaps for all types of metastatic cancer, thoughtful clinical judgement is paramount, recognising that interventions may impose harm even whilst offering symptom relief. Palliation should prioritise quality of life over duration and avoid decisions that merely prolong the process of dying.

Nutritional complications

Malnutrition and cachexia are common in UGI malignancies. In selected patients, enteral feeding via nasogastric or percutaneous endoscopic gastrostomy (PEG) tubes or total parenteral nutrition (TPN) when enteral feeding is not possible may be of value.

Appetite stimulants: Megestrol acetate or corticosteroids may improve intake.

Complications of therapy

Treatments for UGI cancers can cause significant adverse effects.

Chemotherapy-related complications

Chemotherapy can lead to various complications, the commonest being, nausea, vomiting, lack of appetite and oral mucositis. In some dehydration may occur due to diarrhoea, needing hospitalisation and hydration.

Radiotherapy-related complications

- *Oesophagitis:* Sucralfate and analgesics provide symptom relief.
- *Strictures:* Managed with dilatation or stenting.
- *Radiation pneumonitis:* Treated with corticosteroids.

Psychological and social complications

- *Depression and anxiety:* Common in advanced disease; managed with counselling and pharmacotherapy.
- *Caregiver strain:* Support groups and palliative care teams provide relief.

Section 13: Appendix: Key papers on surgical management

There remain controversies in the management of gastric cancers. The extent of the resection of stomach and nodes varies between the Eastern and Western centres.

1. The subtotal versus total gastrectomies
2. D1 versus D2 dissection
3. Hospital volume and surgeon volume
4. Chemoradiotherapy after surgery compared to surgery alone

Subtotal versus total gastrectomies (Figure 5)

Both procedures carry a similar probability of survival provided:

- There is at least 6 cm of clearance from the proximal edge of the tumour to the cardia
- The resection line should not be compromised. Microscopic involvement decreased survival suggesting the need for per operative frozen section (Dutch Gastric Cancer Trial DGCT)
- There is no intraperitoneal spread
- There is no distal spread
- A complete surgical resection is done
- Regional lymphadenectomy is carried out

Hospital mortality rate was, however, much lower after subtotal than total gastrectomy, 3% versus 7% (DGCT). Poorly differentiated cancers may benefit from a total gastrectomy. The subtotal gastrectomy delivers better nutritional status and quality of life.

A total gastrectomy is the therapy of choice for resectable tumours of the proximal and middle stomach. A subtotal gastrectomy is feasible for antral and distal tumours.

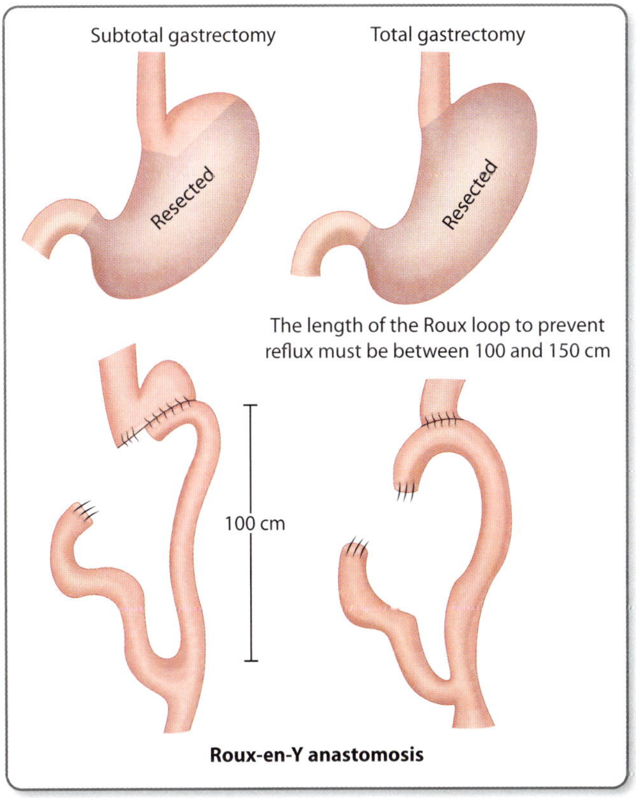

Figure 5 Gastrectomy types and reconstruction.

Resection margin

- *R0 resection:* It is a resection margin that is microscopically and macroscopically negative for malignant cells.
- *R1 resection:* It is a resection that is microscopically positive but macroscopically negative.
- *R2 resection:* It is a resection margin that is microscopically and macroscopically positive.

D1 versus D2 resection

In a D1 dissection (perigastric nodes), a subtotal gastrectomy is carried out along with a 6 cm proximal clearance, resection of the lesser and greater omentum and clearance of the perigastric (N1) nodes.
In a D2 dissection, *N1 and N2 nodes are resected.*

The DGCT and MRC trials showed no significant benefit for D2 dissection over D1 dissection especially in European patients. In Japan where there is screening for gastric cancer, D2 has been the operation of choice.

Volume of surgery

The studies have shown the obvious that where a greater volume of operations is carried out in an institution or by an individual, the results are better — a principle first exemplified by pioneers like Theodor Billroth, the founder of modern abdominal surgery (**Box 1**).

Box 1 Theodor Billroth – the founder of modern abdominal surgery.

Theodor Billroth 1829–1894

Theodor Billroth, a Viennese surgeon, is considered the *father of modern abdominal surgery*. He was *Carl Langenbuch's* (whose retractor we use even today) assistant in Berlin before becoming the professor of surgery in Vienna.

He was an early adopter of the '*white coat*' and introduced *antiseptics* in his clinics as he had a considerable interest in the origin of '*wound fever*'.

In 1881, he performed the first successful 'formidable' distal gastric resection for an antral tumour, on Therese Heller, who lived for almost 4 months and died of liver metastases. The reconstruction he did goes by his name Billroth 1.

Billroth 1 antrectomy and gastroduodenostomy

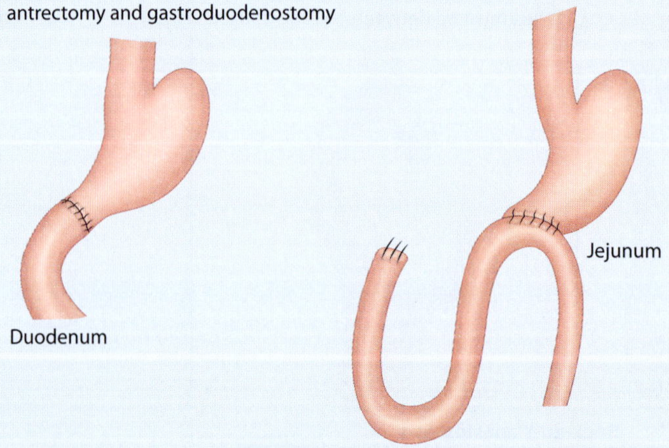

Billroth 2 distal gastrectomy and antecolic gastrojejunostomy

Section 14: Oesophageal cancer

This tends to be either:

- *A squamous cell carcinoma:* Upper and mid oesophagus
- *An adenocarcinoma:* Lower oesophagus

Presenting symptoms

- Dysphagia for solids more than liquids
- Unexplained weight loss
- Persistent dyspepsia
- Retrosternal discomfort

Investigations

These are similar to the oesophago-gastric cancer described above.

Endoscopy and confirmation of histology is needed prior to the initiation of the other investigations.

The purpose of further investigations is to assess the extent of the disease to help to define the appropriate treatment for an individual.

Staging of the disease is dependent on the TNM classification for squamous cell cancers and adenocarcinoma.

TNM staging

Tumour

- *T1* limited to mucosa *(T1a)* and submucosa *(T1b).*
- *T2* cancer involves muscularis propria or muscular layer of the oesophagus.
- *T3* cancer involves serosa
- *T4* cancer involves adjacent organs or body structures next to the oesophagus.
  - *T4a:* Involves pleura, pericardium, peritoneum and diaphragm
  - *T4b:* Involves trachea, vertebra and aorta or blood vessels

Nodes

- *N0:* No lymph nodes involved
- *N1:* 1 or 2 nearby lymph nodes involved
- *N2:* 3–6 nearby lymph nodes involved
- *N3:* 7 or more nearby lymph nodes involved.

Metastasis

- *M0:* No distant organs involved
- *M1:* Spread to distant organs

Treatment

Surgical resection – oesophagectomy or oesophagogastrectomy.

- Oesophagectomy is the standard surgical treatment for resectable oesophageal cancer. This may be by a thoraco-abdominal approach or with minimally invasive techniques.

In some situations, anastomosis may be in the neck. These procedures involve mobilising the stomach and drawing it up into the thorax to enable a tension-free anastomosis.

Three primary approaches dominate clinical practice:

- *Transhiatal oesophagectomy:* This method avoids thoracotomy by combining abdominal and cervical incisions. It is often employed for lower oesophageal tumours.
- *Ivor Lewis oesophagectomy:* A two-stage transthoracic approach incorporating laparotomy and right thoracotomy, allowing optimal exposure for lymphadenectomy and anastomosis.
- *Three-field oesophagectomy:* Includes cervical lymphadenectomy in addition to abdominal and thoracic dissections. While oncologically superior, this method carries higher morbidity and is typically reserved for select cases.
- *EMR* – endoscopic resection may be suitable for in situ lesions in Barrat's and for high-grade dysplasia
- Chemotherapy
- Radiotherapy
- Chemoradiotherapy (chemotherapy together with radiotherapy)
- Targeted or immunotherapy cancer drugs
- Stenting to enable swallowing
- Palliative for control of symptoms

Table 2 shows the 5-year survival rates for oesophageal cancers.

The management of Gastro-oesophageal cancers continues to represent formidable and complex problems with delayed diagnoses, often in elderly and unfit patients. Recognition, of factors such as *H. pylori* infections, GORD and obesity may help in the reduction of risk. As research advances, the integration of molecular profiling, immunotherapy, and improved screening strategies offers hope that the burden of these cancers may be reduced in the decades ahead.

Table 2 The 5-year survival rates for oesophageal cancers.

Extent of involvement	5-year survival
Localised disease	49%
Regional disease	28%
Distant disease	6%
All SEER stages combined	22%

SEER, Surveillance, Epidemiology and End Results.
Source: American Cancer Society SEER database, maintained by National Cancer Institute).

Chapter 5

Small bowel malignancies

Srinivasan Ravi, Ilias Marios Oikonomou, Marena Gray,
Vlasios Gourgiotis, Stavros Gourgiotis

Section 1: Introduction, epidemiology and incidence

The small intestine (SI) is the longest part of the entire digestive tract. It is approximately 6 m in length and four times the length of the large bowel. It has 90% of the absorptive surface area of the gastrointestinal tract (GIT). It is the site of absorption of proteins, lipids, and carbohydrates. It has a very sophisticated system of immune cells that are able to distinguish the non-self from the self. The three parts of the SI are the duodenum, jejunum, and ileum. Despite constituting 75% of the GIT, small bowel malignancies are rare (**Table 1**). When they do occur, their detection is delayed unless fortuitously noted on incidental scans. The rarity of adenocarcinoma of the small bowel may be explained by the short transit time. This decreases exposure to dietary carcinogens and lowers the density of microbiota which convert bile salts into carcinogenic deoxycholic acid (Delaunoit et al., 2005). The other probable hypotheses include rapid turnover of small intestinal epithelium discarding accumulated genetic damage and increased lymphoid tissue allowing increased immune surveillance.

With low numbers of small bowel cancers being detected in the UK annually, the mortality rate tends to be low at 0.7-1/100,000 compared to 30/100,000 for colorectal cancers.

Section 2: Pathology and distribution

The most common location appears to be the duodenum with 36% of the cases whereas the least common is Meckel's diverticulum with <1% of the cases (**Table 2**).

The cells of origin of this disparate group are varied and reflect the histology.

Gastrointestinal stromal tumour or GIST occurs in the stomach and the small bowel and is a type of sarcoma. They arise from the specialised interstitial cells of Cajal. They assist in

Table 1 UK incidence of small bowel cancer.

Total number of cases	1,809
Proportion of all cancers	<1%
Peak age range	80–84 years
Increase since 1990	163%

Source: Cancer Research UK 2023.

Table 2: Summary of the main types of small intestine (SI) malignancies.

Type of cancer	%	Common location	Peak age	5-year survival
Sarcoma including GIST	8	Ileum	65	80%
Adenocarcinoma	30–40	Duodenum	50–70	65%
Neuroendocrine	35–42	Ileum	50–70	90%
Lymphoma	17	Across the GIT	60–70	60% (3 years survival)

GIST, gastrointestinal stromal tumours; GIT, gastrointestinal tract.
Source: Iida et al., 2020.

the neurotransmission of contents by peristalsis. They are referred to as the pacemakers of the GIT.

Adenocarcinomas arise from the glandular cells that line the mucosa. Their prognosis is poor.

Neuroendocrine tumours (NET), as the name implies, arise from the nerve and endocrine tissues scattered all over the GIT. Some of these may secrete a peptide. They are rare tumours. The ones pertaining to SI and GIT are:

- *Carcinoid*
- Pancreatic NET – islet cells

They are classified into:

- Well-differentiated tumours
- Poorly differentiated tumours

Carcinoid tumours of the digestive tract are tumours that secrete serotonin. The liver breaks down serotonin to 5-hydroxy indole acetic acid (*5-HIAA*) which is then excreted in the urine. Its levels in the urine may be an indicator of *carcinoid syndrome*. Typically, increased level of 5-HIAA is a feature of metastatic carcinoid. The main symptoms are flushing of the skin and diarrhoea (CRUK).

Lymphomas of the SI: Gastrointestinal system is the most common site of extra-nodal lymphoma mostly of the non-Hodgkins type. (Ghimire P, Wu GY, Zhu L. Primary gastrointestinal lymphoma. World J Gastroenterol 2011; 17:697–707.)

Section 3: Risk factors and presenting symptoms

The risk factors are:

- *Modifiable:* Diet, obesity, smoking, alcohol and exposure to organic solvents such as working with leather, paints, etc.
- *Non-modifiable* with characteristics that cannot be changed and over which the patient has no control. These include increasing age, gender, more common in males, and hereditary mutation. Familial adenomatous polyposis and Lynch syndrome is associated with small bowel adenocarcinoma. Inflammation due to autoimmune conditions such as inflammatory bowel disease (IBD) (Crohn's and ulcerative colitis) and coeliac disease have been associated with increased risk of SI adenocarcinomas.

Section 4: Presentation, investigation and staging

The signs and symptoms of SI cancers are non-specific in most.

They include irritable bowel-like symptoms with bloating and cramping abdominal pain, dyspepsia, anaemia and fatigue. Occasionally, they may present with gastrointestinal (GI) bleeding. Some patients may present with flushing, diarrhoea and bronchospasm suggesting carcinoid syndrome (mostly in the presence of metastasis).

Investigations and staging

Very often the diagnosis is made during investigations for the presenting symptoms.

- Routine haematology
- Conventional endoscopy
- Double balloon endoscopy
- CT scan
- Wireless capsule endoscopy
- Biochemical markers

Conventional endoscopy is used to diagnose lesions located at the proximal duodenum (gastroscopy) and very distal ileum (colonoscopy).

Double balloon endoscopy is an ingenious procedure that is carried out with an enteroscope with a balloon at its tip and an over tube with another balloon. The enteroscope is pushed into the small bowel and the balloon at its tip is distended to grasp the small bowel. The over scope tube is pushed distally and its balloon distended to grasp the small bowel. The distal scope balloon is then collapsed and the scope pushed further to enable the scope to walk down the small bowel with serial plication. This procedure is indicated in patients with suspected small bowel pathology. It can be used for pathological confirmation by biopsy. It also facilitates marking the tumour site, by tattooing preoperatively for localisation during open or laparoscopic surgery (Sunada et al., 2005).

Capsule endoscopy may be of value in obscure cases that present with non-specific abdominal pain or anaemia. It does not allow tissue biopsy and is contraindicated in patients with small or large bowel occlusion (Cobrin, Pittman and Lewis, 2006).

CT scan will assist in making the diagnosis.

Once a small bowel pathology is suspected, then tests for markers such as *chromogranin A and urinary HIAA* may assist in the definition of the type of lesion. Chromogranin A is a sensitive and specific marker for NETs and a strong indicator of tumour volume and prognosis. However, absence does not exclude a NET.

Lymphomatous lesions can be multiple and may be present at multiple sites in the ileum and jejunum sometimes mimicking Crohn's disease. Adenocarcinomas are normally located at a single site. Sometimes, these lesions can cause small bowel obstruction.

The American Joint Committee on Cancer (AJCC) TNM staging, updated in 2018, is commonly used worldwide to understand the size and aggressiveness of the tumour and aids in the assessment of the prognosis of the disease.

Section 5: Treatment

Adenocarcinomas

Treatment regimens vary based on the type of small bowel cancer and its stage. When the tumour is classified as adenocarcinoma, especially localised, the first-line treatment option would be surgical resection with clearance of at least 5 cm proximal and distal margin (Locher et al., 2018). Resection of the adjoining mesentery and adequate lymph node removal is also required to prevent metastases and in order to determine whether adjuvant therapy is indicated. In the cases where the duodenum is involved with local invasion of the ampulla of Vater, Whipple's procedure (pancreaticoduodenectomy) is recommended (Cloyd, George and Visser, 2016). However, even after the surgery, prognosis and survival remain poor, with a calculated 5-year survival of 20–50% (Khan et al., 2015). Ecker et al. (2015) investigated the efficacy of adjuvant chemotherapy compared to surgery alone in 4,746 patients. They found that patients who received chemotherapy, capecitabine and oxaliplatin (CAPOX) or folinic acid, fluorouracil, and oxaliplatin (FOLFOX), had a statistically significant improved overall survival (OS) to those who only received surgery with a median OS of 63.2 compared to 44.5 ($p < 0.001$) and that appeared to be the case in all stages I–III.

Metastatic disease is far more challenging to treat. The patients present with advanced disease and unpleasant symptoms. The multidisciplinary team (MDT), along with the patient and their family, will decide on the best option, which often includes palliative care. A third of the patients with small bowel adenocarcinoma will develop metastases, mostly due to late presentation, and 20–50% of them are peritoneal metastases (Sakae et al., 2017; Rovers et al., 2017).

Neuroendocrine tumours and lymphomas

Similar to adenocarcinomas, first-line treatment for NETs is surgical resection for symptom alleviation, especially in obstructive cases, and to prevent metastases, despite the tumour being considered indolent in most patients. Local lymph node and mesenteric invasions or metastases should not be overlooked as they can lead to advanced disease. In cases of advanced disease, chemotherapy is recommended after initial surgery has taken place.

The treatment pathway for SI lymphoma appears to be very similar to NETs.

Sarcomas

As mentioned above, small bowel sarcomas are categorised into gastrointestinal stromal tumours (GIST) and non-GIST tumours. Treatment and management regimen, therefore, differ based on the type of sarcoma. The receptor tyrosine kinase (TK) *KIT* proto-oncogene is upregulated in GIST, making TK inhibitors, like imatinib *(Gleevec)* very effective. Therefore, surgery can sometimes be avoided, which is often a pleasant outcome for patients, in consideration that those tumours do not often metastasise to regional lymph nodes.

Summary

In summary, small bowel malignancies encompass a diverse spectrum of pathological entities that present with subtle and non specific clinical symptoms. Diagnosis can be incidental or difficult and delayed due to the inaccessibility of the small intestine.

Chapter 6

Hepatobiliary malignancies

Srinivasan Ravi

Anatomy of the liver

Morphological anatomy (**Figure 1**) based on the external appearance divides the liver into four lobes, the left and right separated by the falciform ligament and the quadrate and caudate lobes. The blood supply is 20% from the hepatic artery and 80% from the portal vein that drains the gut and spleen; the liver acts as the first filter. The portal vein is only about 8 cm long and 13 mm wide. It is formed behind the pancreas by the confluence of the superior and inferior mesenteric veins that drain the small and large intestine. The other tributaries are the splenic and gastric veins. The venous drainage of the liver is to the hepatic vein and then the inferior vena cava (IVC). The portal and venous systems are in intimate contact in the substance of the liver.

Functional anatomy (**Figure 2**) is more utilitarian with the increasing progress in technology that enables various types of resections of the liver for multiple indications such as primary tumours and metastases. It was described by the French anatomist and surgeon *Claude Couinaud*. In this system the liver is divided into *eight segments* as shown below. The caudate lobe remains as segment one. The other segments are divided by the hepatic and portal veins into different independent functional segments that permit segmental resections. Each of these segments has its own inflow and outflow systems. If the resections are done in the correct planes, good haemostasis can be achieved.

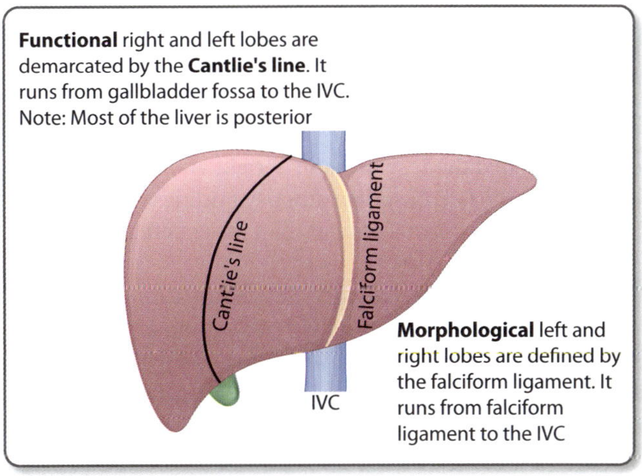

Figure 1 Morphological anatomy. IVC, inferior vena cava.

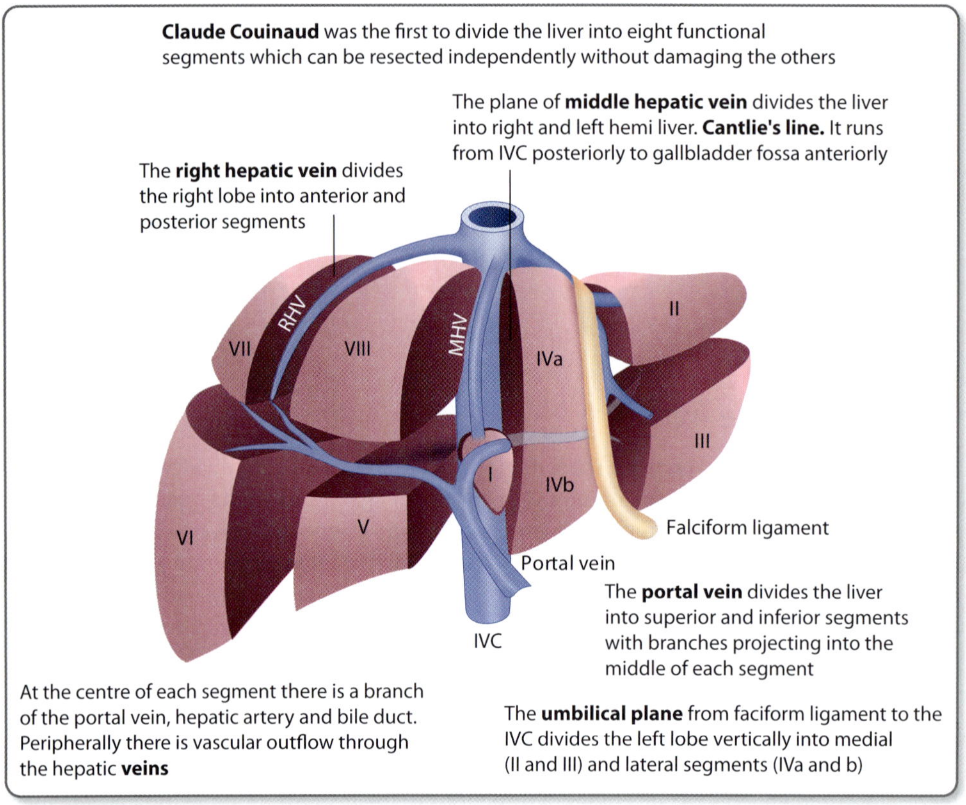

Figure 2 Schematic functional anatomy of the liver.

There are normally three large hepatic veins situated superiorly in the liver draining into the IVC whilst the caudate lobe drains directly into the IVC via several small veins.

- The *right hepatic vein* divides the right lobe into anterior and posterior segments.
- The *middle hepatic vein* lies in the same plane as the IVC and divides the liver into two equal functional segments of left and right hemi liver.
- The *left hepatic vein* (the umbilical plane) according to some divides the left lobe into two vertical segments whilst some anatomists believe that it is the only plane that is not defined by the hepatic or portal veins.
- *The portal vein* (left and right branches) divides the liver into a superior and inferior plane.

Cantlie, a Scottish surgeon, noted, in 1887, that the true division of right and left lobes of the liver was in a plane from the gallbladder to the IVC based on autopsy findings. This plane is useful in hepatectomy and lies lateral to the falciform ligament than the schematic diagram shows (**Figure 1**).

Malignant tumour of the liver can be primary or secondary. Secondary tumours from colorectal cancers are the most common cause of liver tumours. At the time of initial diagnosis 15–20% of colorectal cancer patients may have a liver metastasis with a further 15% going on to develop metachronous disease. Primary liver tumours are more common in Asia and Africa due to increased prevalence of chronic liver disease. Primary liver tumours are:

- Hepatocellular carcinoma
- Cholangiocarcinoma
- Gallbladder carcinoma

Hepatocellular carcinoma

Risk factors:

- *Hepatitis B (HBV) and C (HCV) infections*: Chronic liver disease associated with HBV and HCV is the strongest risk factor globally. A high proportion of cases show evidence of infection with HBV and HCV (Benson et al.).
- *Excessive alcohol intake:* In the UK, alcohol-related cirrhosis is the cause of a third of the liver cancers. Nearly 80% of patients with hepatocellular carcinoma (HCC) have evidence of cirrhosis (Bartlett *DL).*
- *Non-alchoholic fatty liver* [non-alcoholic steatohepatitis (*NASH*)] is now referred to as metabolic dysfunction associated steatotic liver disease (MASLD) related to obesity increasingly thought of as being a risk factor. 20% of cases occur in non-cirrhotic livers.
- *Schistosoma mansoni* is currently thought to be of doubtful significance. It is quite possible that is a co-factor or a promoter in the presence of HBV and HBC infections.
- *Aflatoxin* – long-term exposure increases risk. Aflatoxin is found in grains and peanuts exposed to *Aspergillus* contamination.
- *Rare in born errors of metabolism, haemochromatosis* (build-up of iron), *Wilson's disease* (build-up of copper)

Presentation

This can be very non-specific unless made obvious with jaundice.

- Unexplained weight loss
- Jaundice
- Palpable mass
- Fatigue
- Pyrexia

Pathology

Three gross morphologic types of HCC have been identified:

1. *Nodular* – associated with cirrhosis. Well-circumscribed
2. *Massive* – more common in non-cirrhotic liver. This occupies a large area of the liver
3. *Diffuse* – less common and involves the whole liver

Role of screening

Enrolment in screening in high-risk individuals in China with chronic hepatitis or HBV has shown a benefit. Monitoring of serum alpha fetoprotein (AFP) and ultrasound every 6 months showed a 37% reduction in risk of mortality even when only 60% of the cohort completed the screening programme (Zang). In a separate study in Singapore, screening in high-risk individuals was noted to be of benefit not only in older patients but also in the 40-year-old patients.

Diagnosis

The diagnosis can be challenging as it is mostly insidious. When suspected the primary screening modality is an ultrasound examination of the liver along with routine blood counts, renal and liver function tests including lactate dehydrogenase (LDH), alkaline phosphatase (ALP), albumin, international normalised ratio (INR) and AFP levels.

Alpha fetoprotein: In the presence of an ultrasound detected mass in the liver that is >2 cm an elevated AFP > 200 ng/mL is diagnostic of the HCC. AFP > 200 ng/mL has a specificity of nearly 100% in the presence of chronic liver disease. It must also be noted that AFP may not be elevated in up to 40% of patients with hepatocellular carcinoma, a group referred to as N-HCC. In A-HCC the AFP is raised.

Role of fine-needle biopsy

Fine-needle biopsy (FNB) is associated with problems, such as tumour seeding, which are probably underestimated (Torzilli). The actual risks of FNB and its impact on patient prognosis due to tumour seeding are still unclear.

When the AFP is non-diagnostic preoperative FNB may play a diagnostic role in selected patients with:

- Focal lesions in cirrhotic livers that are indeterminate on imaging
- Focal lesions in non-cirrhotic livers to differentiate from metastatic disease

Any attempt to do a biopsy should be discussed with a specialist liver unit first.

Modalities of radiological imaging are:

- Triphasic helical CT
- Triphasic dynamic contrast-enhanced MRI
- Contrast-enhanced ultrasonography

Triphasic CT involves three phases:

1. *Arterial phase:* This occurs in the first 15–30 seconds after contrast injection.
2. *Portal venous phase* is when the portal vein (80% of oxygenated blood supply) perfuses the lesion a little later than the arterial phase.
3. *Delayed phase: Wash out phase.* This is the phase, 2–5 minutes following contrast.

Typically, in HCC, there is prominence of the tumour with the arterial flush (enhancement) followed by a wash out in the delayed venous phase. In *liver cysts,* there is no enhancement in any of the phases while in *haemangioma,* there is prominence in the arterial and portal venous phases.

Management

This is determined by the:

- Hepatic function
- TNM staging
- Degree of portal hypertension
- Patient's performance status

Surgical resection is the treatment of choice in selected patients.

Surgery depends on:

- The extent of the disease such as limited to the liver
- Resectability of the lesion

- *Adequacy of functional liver remnant (FLR)*
- *Feasibility of a clear resection margin*
- Adequate hepatic function (Child–Pugh score A)
- Absence of signs of portal hypertension. A platelet count of <1,00,000/μL is a very good surrogate for clinically significant portal hypertension
- Absence of metastasis (lungs, abdominal nodes, and bones)

Surgical interventions:
Surgical resection can achieve 5-year survival rates of 60% with a operative mortality of 2–3% in selected patients. Adjuvant systemic immunotherapy may reduce tumour recurrence

- *Downstaging strategies:*
  - *Transarterial chemoembolisation (TACE)*: This treatment utilises the fact that the major blood supply to an HCC is via the hepatic artery whilst the normal liver is mainly supplied by the portal vein. The procedure is performed through a femoral artery access with a catheter that is guided to the tumour via the hepatic artery. It is the most common treatment for unresectable disease and can be used as a bridging therapy for patients awaiting liver transplant.
- *Partial hepatectomy:* Where the disease is localised to a resectable area without invasion of major vascular structures.
- Percutaneous and laparoscopic ablation
- Minimally invasive operations, laparoscopic and robotic surgery
- Parenchyma sparing resection with ultrasound guidance
- Staged hepatectomy
- *Liver transplantation:* The major limitation to this is organ shortage and prolonged waiting times

Radiofrequency ablation (RFA): In situations where resection is not possible or when the tumour is so small that resection can be avoided, percutaneous radiofrequency or microwave ablation can be carried out (CRUK). This works of the principle of using heat to destroy cancer cells akin to diathermy. The area destroyed is limited to the immediate surroundings and the procedure is done by passing a needle through the skin and locating it within the lesion under ultrasound control. Microwave can also be used instead of radiofrequency.

Stereotactic ablative radiotherapy (SABR): This is an alternative modality of treatment using focussed high-dose radiotherapy to destroy liver lesions where surgery is not an option.

Histotripsy: It is a noninvasive ultrasound based therapy that uses high intensity pulsed and focused ultrasound to mechanically destroy tumour tissue in the liver. Focussed ultrasound creates microbubbles (cavitation) which expand and collapse creating 'liquefaction'. Most patients are treated on a day case basis with a single sitting of 1 to 3 hours. Once the tumour is liquified, the immune system does the clearance. This treatment has been approved by the NHS. Further studies are needed assess the complete clearance and side effects such as further spread. Bleeding is a complication. Early results are promising with regard to local control. Long term studies are awaited.

Systemic therapy with tyrosine kinase inhibitors (TKI) such as sorafenib and lenvatinib that disrupt the intracellular pathways leading to cell destruction can be used in situations where surgical treatment cannot be offered (CRUK).

Liver transplant in hepatocellular carcinoma

Liver transplant can be used in selected patients where the tumour burden is small. It improves outcome in otherwise non-resectable lesions with cirrhosis.

Milan criteria for liver transplant was introduced in 1996 by Mazzaferro et al. The criteria are considered restrictive by some.

- A single tumour with a diameter of <5 cm
- Up to three tumours, each with a diameter of <3 cm
- No evidence of extrahepatic spread
- No evidence of macrovascular invasion

Child–Pugh score (ABCDE)

This scoring system gives an indication of the liver function and it classifies the severity of cirrhosis of the liver. It is, therefore, used to predict mortality in cirrhotic patients.

- A = Albumin level
- B = Bilirubin
- C = Coagulation – INR
- D = Deluge – ascites
- E = Hepatic encephalopathy

The Child–Pugh scoring system is from A to C, with C indicating the worst hepatic function.

Each factor is given points (1, 2, or 3) based on its severity.

- *Class A*: 5–6 points (well-compensated)
- *Class B*: 7–9 points (moderately decompensated)
- *Class C*: 10–15 points (significantly decompensated)

Cholangiocarcinoma

These are uncommon cancers. There are two types.

1. Intrahepatic cholangiocarcinoma
2. Extrahepatic cholangiocarcinoma

These can be:

- Perihilar *(Klatskin tumour)*
- Distal bile duct carcinoma

The presentation is normally with jaundice and unexplained weight loss.

Diagnosis is made with routine blood tests and liver function tests that show jaundice. *CEA and CA19-9* may be elevated.

Primary sclerosing cholangitis must be excluded.

Investigations may include:

- Endoscopic retrograde cholangiopancreatography (ERCP)
- *Endoscopic ultrasound examination (EUS):* This can also be used to get cytology.

Radiological investigations include CT scan, MRCP, and MRI.

- *Percutaneous transhepatic cholangiogram (PTC)* may be needed in select cases where access is not possible via ERCP.

Treatment

Treatment is in specialised liver units.

It depends on the:

- Location
- Invasion
- Extent and spread

Very often these cancers are detected late and only *palliative treatment* may be feasible.

Gallbladder carcinoma

These, like the cholangiocarcinoma, are rare cancers that are seldom detected early. The presentation and work-up is similar to that of the cholangio carcinoma or chronic cholecystitis. Early-stage cancers that are limited to the gallbladder can be removed laparoscopically. Curative surgery is seldom possible when the cancer has spread beyond the confines of the gallbladder. Newer modalities of immunotherapy and targeted chemotherapy are currently being developed and studied.

Pancreatic malignancies

Gross anatomy of pancreas (Figure 3)

Pancreatic cancer (**Figure 4**) is the 10th most common cancer in the UK.

Presentation may be subtle and often missed in the early stages.

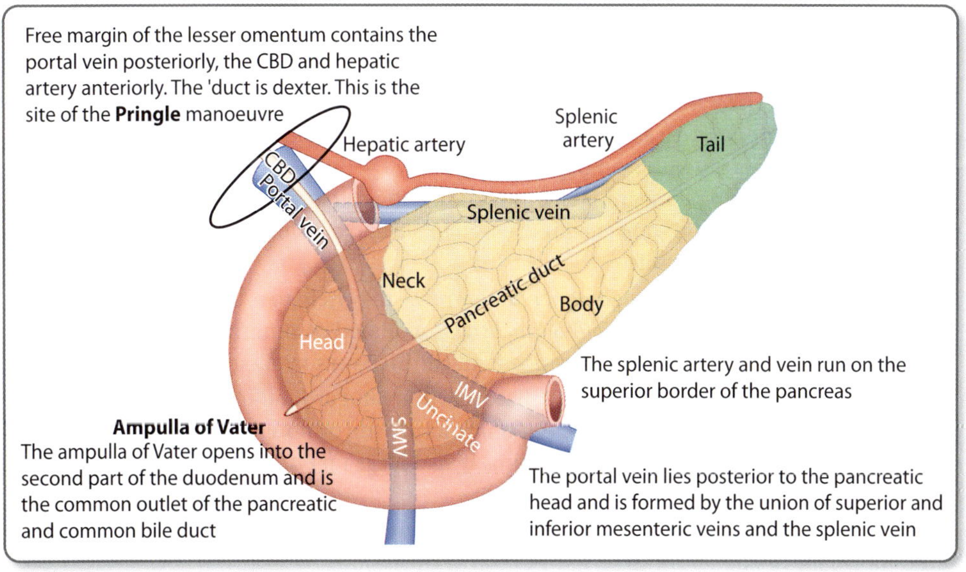

Figure 3 Anatomy of the pancreas.

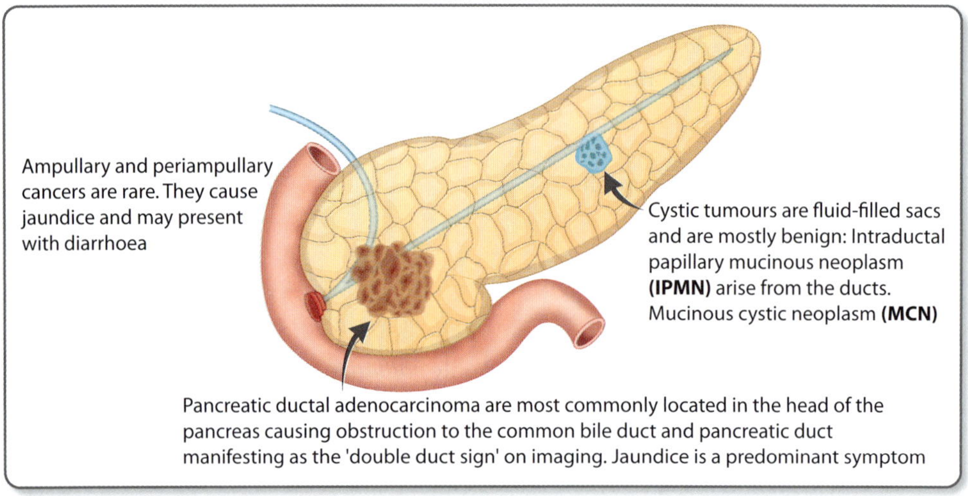

Figure 4 Exocrine pancreatic tumours.

Commonly it presents as:

- Painless progressive jaundice (obstructive)
- Pruritus
- Unexplained weight loss
- Diarrhoea
- Back pain
- Evidence of deep vein thrombosis (DVT) – migratory thrombophlebitis. Trousseau's sign of malignancy. This is a para neoplastic syndome, presenting mostly with migratory superficial and tender thrombosis, presenting as phlebitis.

In patients with obstructive jaundice, the liver function test will be grossly abnormal with an elevated ALP.

Tumour markers CA-19-9 (commonly found in the biliary system and is elevated in acute and chronic biliary disease and pancreatic cancers) and CEA may be raised.

Investigations are done to assess suitability for curative or palliative treatment and to aid in confirming the diagnosis with cytology or biopsy.

- *Endoscopy* may often be the initial investigation if the cause of the weight loss is unclear. In some situations, if the scope can be passed to D2 and a lesion noted, a biopsy for tissue diagnosis is invaluable
- *Endoscopic retrograde cholangiopancreatography* – may help to establish the diagnosis with a biopsy. Classically, the *double-duct sign* – a dilated common bile duct and a pancreatic duct may be seen on diagnostic ERCP. Biopsy or cytology can be carried out.
- *CT scan* – will define the extent of the disease within and around the pancreas. A triple phase of CT scan is used as this will not only pick up the tumour but also define its relationship to the main arteries and veins. It also picks up *pancreatic cysts.* Not all pancreatic cysts are malignant.
- *MRI or MRCP* of the pancreas will assist in clarifying the nature of the pathology. This is not normally needed but can be used to clarify the lesion.

- *PET-CT* – This is done to quantify the total disease load and the presence of metastasis.
- *Endoscopic ultrasound (EUS):* This is of increasing value as it allows for ultrasound examination in close proximity to the pancreas. It helps to define cysts, aspirate tissue for cytology.

Pancreatic cysts

- *Intraductal papillary mucinous neoplasms (IPMN):* These arise in the ducts and secrete mucous thus forming a cyst. Depending upon the number of high-risk features such as duct size and the presence of nodules the risk of developing malignancy in main duct IPMN is 70% and for side-branch ducts is 20%.
- *Mucinous cyst neoplasms (MCN):* These arise in the body and tail of the pancreas and can turn malignant.
- *Serous cystadenoma (SCA):* These are non-cancerous and can be found anywhere in the pancreas.

Differentiating between mucinous and serous cystadenomas is important as the former has a malignant potential. The mucinous cystadenomas are larger cysts with calcification in the circumference, 'egg shell calcification'. The serous adenomas have a central stellate calcification and are microcystic. Density differences, measured in Hounsfield units, on CT scan can differentiate between these two but are thought to be unreliable.

Treatment

As always it depends on:

- The extent of the disease as quantified by TNM (**Table 1**)
- Nutritional status of the patient
- Suitability for surgery

Table 1 TNM category.

Category	Description
T1	Tumour 2 cm or less
T2	Tumour 2–4 cm
T3	Tumour larger than 4 cm but within pancreas
T4	Tumour involves adjacent structures/blood vessels
N0	No affected nodes
N1	1–3 nodes involved
N2	Four or more nodes involved
M0	No metastasis
M1	Presence of metastases

Surgery

Resection of part or whole of the pancreas may be carried out when a curative resection, that is possible in only about 20% of the patients can be carried out. The most common surgical operation for a resection of a tumour in the pancreatic head is a *pylorus preserving technique.*

The classical operation should probably be called *the Kausch–Whipple pancreatoduodenectomy* as Walther Kausch, a German surgeon, first described a significant resection of the duodenum and pancreas in 1909 and *Allen Whipple,* an American surgeon, subsequently reported three resectional cases in 1935.

The Whipple's operation can be a massive undertaking and fraught with complications including a prolonged recovery. The principle of the operation involves resection of the malignant tumour in the pancreatic head with satisfactory clearance and reconstruction either through open, laparoscopic or robotic-assisted surgery.

The resection, apart from the lesion includes:

- Distal stomach
- Duodenum
- Common bile duct and gallbladder
- Adjacent lymph glands

Reconstruction is done with:

- Gastrojejunostomy – this may be done using a Roux-en-Y loop of jejunum
- Choledochojejunostomy
- Pancreaticojejunostomy

A modified operation with preservation of the pylorus is increasingly more commonly performed.

If the tumour is located distally, a distal pancreatectomy may be carried out.

Extended resections (Fortner operation types 1 and 2)

Where a cancer in the head of the pancreas is encroaching upon adjacent major vessels a superior mesenteric artery (SMA)-first approach can be used. To obtain clear margins a segment of portal vein can be resected with the tumour followed by an end-to-end anastomosis. Rarely part of the SMA can be taken and the artery re-anastomosed with or without a vein graft.

- *Type 1:* Includes resection of the pancreatic segment of the portal vein followed by end-to-end anastomosis *without a graft.*
- *Type 2:* Along with a type 1 resection, this includes resection of the involved artery most often either the hepatic or superior mesenteric artery. A primary arterial anastomosis can be carried out; where that is not feasible, a vein graft can be used.

These are major operations and carry a high risk of mortality and morbidity. Careful assessment and discussions of the risks and benefits with the patient and surrogates are needed.

Multimodality treatment: Chemotherapy alone and with radiotherapy can be given to patients prior to surgery in the form of neoadjuvant therapy if the primary tumour is considered borderline resectable due to involvement of major vessels. This may help achieve negative resection margins.

Adjuvant chemotherapy given after surgery is now the standard of care and has been shown to improve overall survival at 5 years from under 10% to nearly 30% (ESPAC-4 trial, Lancet, 389, 1011, 2017).

Surveillance

The National Institute for Health and Care Excellence (NICE) recommends monitoring for pancreatic cancer in patients with:

- *Hereditary pancreatitis* with a fault in *PRSS1* gene
- *Peutz-Jegers syndrome:* There is a greater risk of bowel and breast cancer but also a risk for pancreatic cancer.
- *Two or more first-degree relatives* with pancreatic cancer, across two or more generations
- *Lynch syndrome and any first-degree* relatives with pancreatic cancer

Palliation

Unfortunately, many patients present late in the disease and palliative operations or treatment alone may be possible. The advent of ERCP has enabled stenting of the common bile duct to relieve the jaundice and pruritus and improve the quality of residual life which in many cases may only be a few months.

In patients with predominantly gastric outlet obstruction syndrome a gastro-jejunostomy anterior to the transverse colon may help to relieve the symptoms.

Chemoradiotherapy prior to surgery can be used to downstage the disease. More often than not, these are used for palliation to prolong life which must be balanced with the quality of residual life.

Survival rates in pancreatic cancer (Table 2)

Unfortunately most patients with pancreatic cancer present with late stage disease and efforts are required for earlier diagnosis. This is based on statistics from a study which included over 35,000 people diagnosed with pancreatic cancer in seven countries. These included Australia, Canada, Denmark, Ireland, New Zealand, Norway, and the UK. British Journal of Cancer, March 2022, Volume 126, pages 1774–82.

Table 2 Survival rates in pancreatic cancer at different stages.

Stages	Survival rate
Localised	55% survive 1 year 25% survive 3 years
Regional	50% survive 1 year 15% survive 3 years
Distant	10% survive 1 year 1% survive 3 years

Conclusion

Surgical resection remains the only potentially curative treatment for carcinoma of the pancreas, but it is feasible in only a small proportion of patients. Even in carefully selected cases, major pancreatic resections are technically demanding and associated with significant morbidity. Owing to the aggressive nature of the disease and its tendency for late presentation, the majority of patients are unsuitable for curative surgery at diagnosis. As a result, treatment in most cases is palliative, aimed at relieving symptoms and improving quality of life rather than achieving cure.

Chapter 7

Colo-rectal disease

Srinivasan Ravi

Section 1: Gross anatomy of the large bowel (Figure 1)

The large bowel extends from the ileocecal valve to the anus and measures 120–150 cm in adults. The cecum, the most proximal saccular part of the large bowel, lies inferior to a horizontal line defined by the ileocecal valve. The cecum is *completely invested by peritoneum* and contains the opening of the vermiform appendix. The right colon, 15–20 cm in length, extends to the hepatic flexure. The right colon lacks mesentery and lies mostly in the retroperitoneum. The transverse colon runs from the hepatic flexure to the splenic flexure, and has a mesentery. The descending colon begins at the splenic

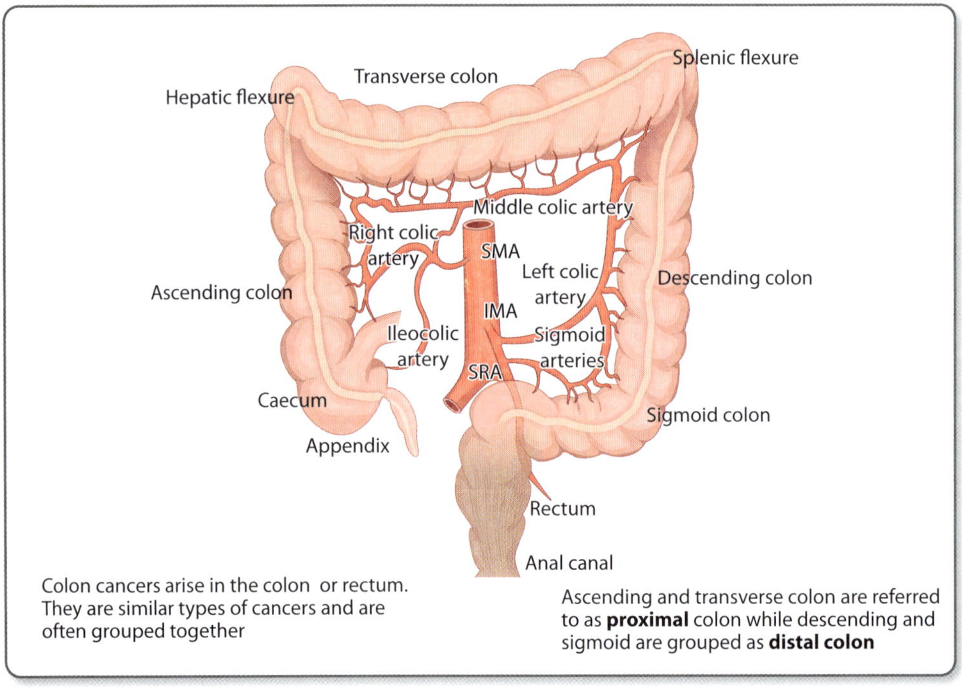

Figure 1 Anatomy of the colon.

SMA, superior mesenteric artery; IMA, inferior mesenteric artery; SRA, superior rectal artery.

flexure, becomes retroperitoneal, and extends for 20–25 cm. More distally, the large bowel acquires a mesentery to become the sigmoid colon. The sigmoid colon arbitrarily becomes the rectum at approximately the level of the third sacral vertebra. The rectum, measuring 10–15 cm in length, ends at the anal canal. The upper one-third of the rectum is covered by peritoneum; the lower two-thirds lies in the retroperitoneum surrounded by the fatty mesorectum.

The colon (**Figure 1**) has mucosal, submucosal and serosal layers. There is an inner circular muscle layer and an outer longitudinal layer. *Taenia coli* are three longitudinal strips of smooth muscle about 6–10 mm in width. They envelope the circular muscle layer. They run from the caecum to the sigmoid and merge with the longitudinal layer of the rectum which has *no Taenia coli*. As they are shorter than the length of the colon, they are thought to be responsible for causing sacculations called haustra that are typical of the colon.

Paracolic gutters are spaces beside the ascending and descending colon that direct inflammatory collections towards the pelvis and elsewhere within the peritoneal cavity. These embryological folds are avascular planes that aid dissection when there is no pathology. However, pathological planes can be adherent and vascular, making dissections more difficult.

The superior mesenteric artery supplies the caecum, ascending colon, and proximal two-thirds of the transverse colon, which are derivatives of the midgut. The rest of the colon is supplied by the inferior mesenteric artery. Similarly, venous drainage flows into the superior and inferior mesenteric veins, part of the *portal system*. This explains why metastatic colorectal cancers, often spread to the liver, which serves as the first filter.

The marginal artery of Drummond is formed by a chain of anastomoses of the terminal branches of the arteries supplying the colon. This permits a good collateral supply to the whole colon. Arising from the marginal arteries, are straight arteries called vasa recta that finally supply the colon. *Griffiths' point* is a critical point at the splenic flexure where marginal branches of the superior mesenteric artery and the marginal artery branch of the inferior mesenteric artery supply the descending colon. Arteriographic studies show the presence of arterial anastomosis between the branches at Griffith's point in 48%, none in 43% and poor in 9%. This point is significant after surgical ligation of the inferior mesenteric artery, as individuals without reliable arterial anastamoses are vulnerable to low perfusion states, potentially leading to ischaemic colitis or ischaemia of the proximal left colon.

The arterial supply to the distal colon is from the inferior mesenteric artery that splits into the left colic and then the sigmoid and superior rectal vessels. During dissection there is a clear avascular space in the mesentery just distal to the left colic branch allowing for ligation of the inferior mesenteric artery at this level. There is ongoing debate about the difference between high and low tie of the inferior mesenteric artery while carrying out anterior resection. Many meta-analyses have been carried out with conflicting results. Most suggest that there is no difference between ligation of the inferior mesenteric artery proximal to the left colic artery (high tie) and distal to the left colic artery. The author prefers the low tie as in theory at least a good blood supply to the left colon should protect the anastomosis and there has been no suggestion that there is a difference in the survival rates between these two approaches.

Table 1 Lifetime risk of colorectal cancer (Houlston et al., 1990).	
Risk to the general population	1 in 50
One affected first-degree relative – *any* age	1 in 17
One affected first and one second-degree relative	1 in 12
One affected first-degree relative *under* the age of 45 years	1 in 10
Two affected first-degree relatives	1 in 6
Autosomal dominant pedigree	1 in 2

Section 2: Risk factors and genetic syndromes (Table 1)

Most colorectal cancers (CRC), however, arise sporadically but can be familial or inherited. When inherited, there is generally a genetic mutation, driving the cancer. Familial cancers may not have a genetic basis.

- *Sporadic* cancers arise randomly
- *Familial* cancers run in families
- *Inherited* cancers occur due to genetic defects such as familial adenomatosis polyposis, hereditary non-polyposis colon cancer or Lynch syndrome, etc.

Specific germline mutations are responsible for inherited CRC. Stepwise accumulation of somatic mutations underlies most sporadic cases of CRC.

Hereditary non-polyposis colon cancer (HNPCC) is the most common form of inherited CRC. Approximately 2–4% of CRC are due to HNPCC. It is defined clinically if the patient satisfies the Amsterdam criteria.

HNPCC and Lynch syndrome refer to the same inherited cancer predisposition syndrome. 'Lynch syndrome' is the preferred and more commonly used term today, as it better reflects the broader spectrum of associated cancers beyond colorectal cancer, including endometrial, ovarian, gastric, small bowel, hepatobiliary, urinary tract, and others.

Lynch syndrome is fundamentally an MMR-defect syndrome, its genetic basis includes classical *MMR* gene mutations. In this group, there is an 80% risk of CRC in adults aged 70 years and above compared to general population risk of 2% by that age without the mutation (Cleveland Clinic).

Modified Amsterdam criteria

The clinical criteria to be met to diagnose HNPCC is referred to as the Amsterdam criteria.

To meet the Amsterdam Criteria for HNPCC (Lynch syndrome) the requirements are:

- At least three relatives with HNPCC associated cancers, one being a first degree relative of the other two
- Involvement of at least two successive generations
- At least one diagnosis before the age of 50
- Colorectal cancer can be replaced by endometrial cancer or small bowel adenocarcinoma
- Familial adenomatous polyposis must be excluded
- All tumours must be confirmed histopathologically

Henry T Lynch noted these familial clusters of cancer and reported several families in detail in 1966–1967. Lynch was aware of Warthin's 'Cancer Family G'. (Warthin, a pathologist, had noted families with colon cancers in 1913).

Lynch conducted a detailed medical genetic investigation of the family G and obtained data on >650 family members (among whom 95 had now developed cancers), and found a predominance of cancers of the colon, uterus and stomach in the kindred (The iconic 'Cancer Family "G" Revisited' manuscript of 1971). Progeny of affected individuals continued to be at risk for early-onset cancers.

He recognised the autosomal dominant nature of inheritance. The time for discovery of the basis of hereditary cancer had not yet arrived and these were thought to be environmental cancers. He used the term 'Cancer Family Syndrome'.

Dr Lynch continued his research, but his theories were widely discredited until molecular genetics techniques developed in the 1980s led to the discovery of the mismatch repair gene deficiencies and associated microsatellite instabilities found in these heritable cancers. HNPCC was renamed Lynch syndrome in his honour in 1984.

Dr Lynch is credited with facilitating many breakthroughs in cancer genetics, including identifying the breast-ovarian cancer syndrome and the *BRCA* genes and creating the entire field of cancer genomics.

(Based on PMC: History of Lynch Syndrome)

Familial adenomatous *Polyposis coli*

This is an inherited autosomal dominant condition that eventually inevitably leads to carcinoma of the colon in the affected individuals. It accounts for <1% of CRC in the West, where CRC rates are higher than in Asia. (*Orphanet- ORPHA : 733 Familial adenomatous polyposis*)

The predominant genetic abnormality is a germline mutation in the *APC* gene.

This leads to formation of myriads of polyps in the colon often numbering in 100s or more in the affected population.

- The presentation can be as early as in their teens with rectal bleeding or anaemia
- *Extracolonic manifestations:*
  - Osteomas
  - Dental abnormalities
  - Extracolonic cancers of thyroid, liver, central nervous system (CNS) or rarely duodenum
  - Presence of congenital hypertrophy retinal pigment epithelium – CHIRPE

The management is based on the family history and clinical findings. The confirmation requires a colonoscopy with genetic testing.

Surgical management with prophylactic total proctocolectomy leads to a 100% prevention when done in the late teens or early 20s. If rectum is preserved with ileo-rectal anastomosis, then the rectum should be screened at regular intervals.

Section 3: Role of genes in colorectal cancers

Molecular basis of CRC tumourigenesis

Major abnormalities are found in:

- Oncogenes – stimulate cell growth to make it hyperactive
- Tumour suppressor genes – such as *APC* and *p53*
- Mismatch repair genes (*MMR*) genes

Oncogenes

Oncogenes are mutated genes that drive malignancy.

Most implicated oncogene is the *RAS*. K-ras is a protein that relays messages from the cell membrane to the nucleus. It controls cell growth, maturation and death. The gene that produces k-ras protein is a *proto-oncogene called 'KRAS,'* meaning that this is a normal gene that has mutated to become an oncogene, a gene that promotes growth (accelerator). *p53*, for example, is a suppressor gene (brake).

There are three variants of the RAS family of oncogenes.

1. *HRAS*
2. *KRAS*
3. *NRAS*

KRAS is the most frequently mutated gene in CRC. When mutated, they have the potential to cause cancer. These mutations are referred to as 'gain of function' mutation as it results in uncontrolled cellular proliferation (accelerator). The importance of *RAS* is underscored by the finding that CRC cells in which a mutated *RAS* gene has been removed or replaced lose their ability to form tumours in nude mice. *RAS* mutations are found in up to 50% of CRCs and adenomas larger than 1 cm. They are rarely seen in smaller adenomas suggesting that *RAS* mutations are acquired during later progression of an adenoma. It must be noted, however, that *RAS* mutations are also noted in about 25% of hyperplastic polyps. The significance of this is unclear at present.

APC suppressor gene

- Perhaps the most critical suppressor gene in the early development of CRC
- Somatic mutations in both alleles are present in 80% of sporadic CRCs
- *A single germline mutation in this gene is responsible for FAP. APC gene is mutated in 100% of FAP patients.*

Adenomatous polyposis coli gene or *APC* gene, when mutated, pushes the cell towards malignancy by its sustained action on cell proliferation and inhibition of differentiation. The predominant predictor of change is TIME. Given time, most genetic mutations multiply. That is also the reason why malignancies are more common in the elderly.

The *p53* gene (Figure 2)

The *p53* gene is located on chromosome 17 and is the most commonly mutated gene in human cancers. 17p sequences are lost in 75% of CRCs while they are rarely lost in adenomas and aberrant crypt foci suggesting that *p53* loss represents a relatively late event in colorectal tumourigenesis.

Figure 2 Polyp – cancer progression.

Polyp cancer genetic sequence
Accumulated genetic defects

APC gene mutation
(Lack of suppression)
Initiation of tumour
KRAS mutation
Many other genetic mutations
p53 mutation in at least 75%
Adenocarcinoma

p53 is the *guardian of the genome* (**Figure 2**) and an important gene involved in apoptosis. It stops the cell cycle and allows cells with mismatched sequence to be repaired by mismatch repair (*MMR*) genes. If it fails, it induces apoptosis or cell death. It stands to reason, therefore, that upregulation of *p53* in response to DNA damage due to radiation or sun rays, is beneficial if the *p53* is normal. *Mutation in p53* prevents its normal function and leads to transmission of errors that permits cancer cells to multiply instead of committing suicide or apoptosis. *In almost all cancers mutations in p53 are noted.*

Section 4: Polyps and polypcancer sequence

A polyp is a protrusion of an aggregation of cells that pile up high on the mucosal surface. Possibly as much as 95% of CRC arise from polyps. They are classified on the basis of their appearance, histology or size (**Figure 3**).

Appearance

- Pedunculated
- Sessile
- Depressed
- Flat

Histology

- Adenomatous: 70–80%
- Villous: 5–15%
- Tubulo villous: 5–15%
- Serrated
- Hyperplastic (non-neoplastic)

Size

- Diminutive <5 mm
- Small: <1 cm
- Large: >1 cm

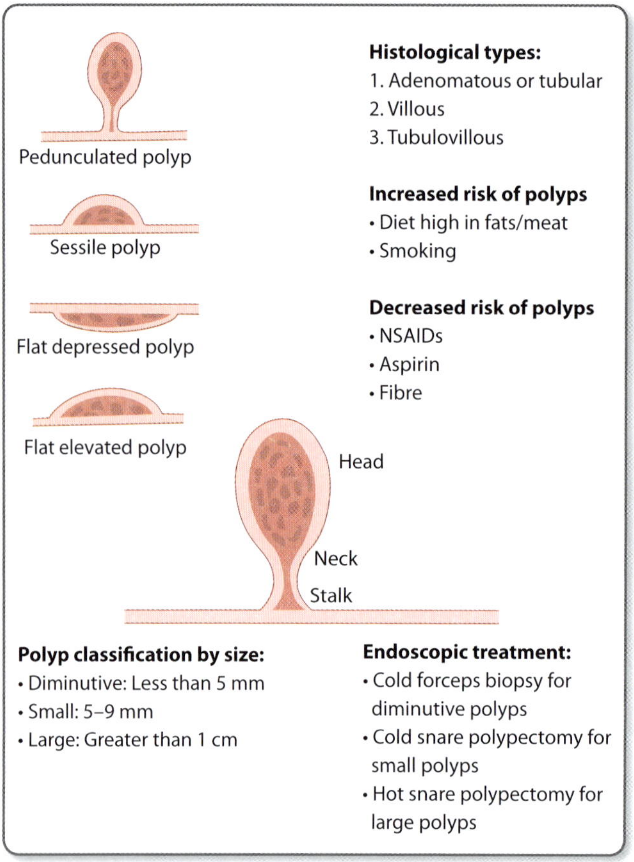

Figure 3 Paris classification of polyps by appearance.

Polyp cancer epithelial sequence

Hyperplasia – low-grade dysplasia – high-grade dysplasia – adenocarcinoma

The polyps progress in size and with dysplasia that occurs with changes in the genetic structure. In the late 1980s, Fearon and Vogelstein described CRC as a genetic disease, with the polyp-to-carcinoma progression as a sequence of specific genetic mutations. The process of piling up starts with the number of cells increasing but (*hyperplasia*) contained by the basement membrane. As they pile high, they become disorderly. This is called *dysplasia*. Changes start occurring in the cell nucleus and the disorder increases. Depending on the nature and number of the dysplastic cells the changes are regarded as *low- and high-grade dysplasia*. The greater the dysplasia, the higher the chance of a malignant change which is the penetration of the basement membrane by the dysplastic cells.

Polyps may progress over time to cancers (but not all do). There is evidence to suggest that this may be the case as we find:

- Polyps adjacent to bowel cancers in a large proportion of cases when reviewing the histology
- Early carcinomas are frequently seen within large adenomatous polyps
- Areas of adenomatous change can often be found surrounding human CRCs

- Adenomas and carcinomas are found in similar distributions throughout the large bowel
- The ability to reduce the incidence of subsequent CRC through removal of polyps has been shown in controlled trials in humans

- Evidence has been presented to show that most carcinomas of the large bowel develop in an adenoma, and that the life history of this sequence, although variable, probably takes on average 10–15 years. However, when the absolute numbers of adenomas and carcinomas are compared, it is apparent that the transition is uncommon. On a statistical analysis, the malignant potential of adenomas is related to their size, growth pattern, and degree of epithelial atypia.
- Recently several studies have demonstrated that CRC screening and removal of precancerous colon adenomas leads to a reduction in CRC incidence and mortality by approximately 50%.
- A natural history study of unresected colonic polyps greater than 1 cm in size in patients who declined surgical resection reported a 24% risk of invasive adenocarcinoma at the site of the index polyp and a 35% risk of carcinoma at any colonic site after 20 years.

- Adenomas are typically observed 10–15 years prior to onset of cancer in sporadic/familial cases

Large polyps may progress to cancer as they acquire more and more mutations. The Fearon–Vogelstein model (**Figure 4**) suggests that cancers progress with a series of mutations from normal cells to cancer cells. It is now recognised that there may be other models and that some cancers may develop along different genetic pathways (Ilyas and Tomlinson).

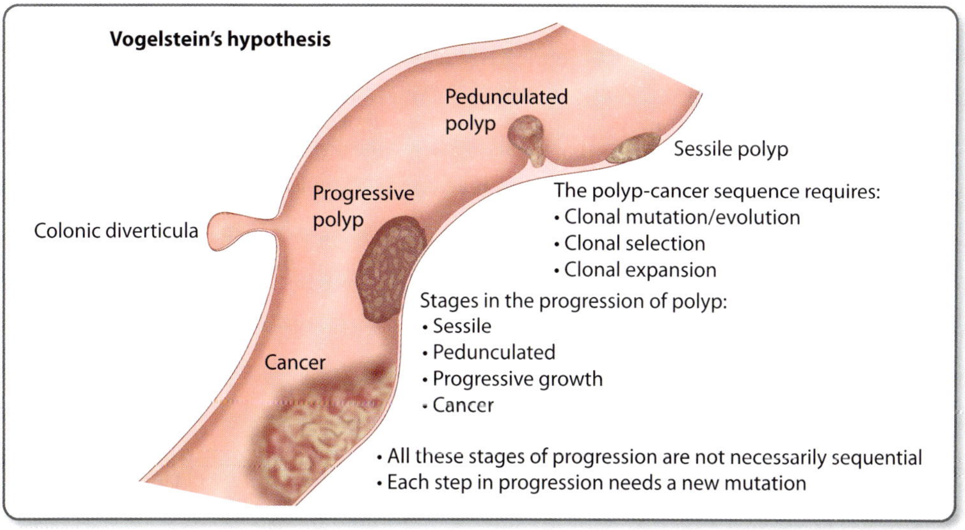

Figure 4 Polyp-cancer sequence.

Table 2 Haggitt levels are used for pedunculated polyps.	
Levels	Description
1	Carcinoma limited to the head of the polyp
2	Carcinoma invading the neck of the polyp
3	Carcinoma invading the stalk of the polyp
4	Carcinoma invading the bowel wall below the stalk but above the muscularis propria. This is considered to be an invasive carcinoma

Table 3 Application of Kikuchi levels for the depth of submucosal penetration in sessile/depressed polyps.	
Level	Description
SM1	Tumour invades upper third of the submucosa
SM2	Tumour invades the middle third of the submucosa
SM3	Tumour invades the lower third of the submucosa
SM, submucosal.	

Polyps can be removed by a number of methods and subjected to histological scrutiny.

Most commonly they can be removed:
Endoscopically:

- Standard snare polypectomy
- Endoscopic mucosal resection (EMR)
- Endoscopic submucosal dissection (ESD)
- *Surgically* (rectal polyps under anaesthesia)
- Transanal endoscopic microsurgery (TEMS)
- Transanal minimally invasive surgery (TAMIS)

Malignant polyps are classified as T1 in the TNM classification.

Histological scrutiny will assess the depth of invasion to help to determine the prognosis or the need for further treatment. This process is dependent on the completeness and intact removal of the polyp. Haggitt and Kikuchi levels are used for staging pedunculated and sessile polyps. The lymph nodal involvement is as low as 3% in Haggitt level 1 but may be as high as 25% in Haggitt level 4 (**Table 2**).

Kikuchi levels are used for *sessile and depressed polyps.* It judges the level of penetration of the submucosa (**Table 3**).

Section 5: Bowel cancer screening

Faecal immunochemical test

The faecal immunochemical test (FIT) is used as a screening test for bowel cancer in the UK. It tests for faecal Hb (occult) in the stools. FIT only detects *human* blood from the lower intestines (**Table 4**).

Table 4 The cancer detection rate.

Faecal Hb level	Positivity for CRC
fHb below 4 µg Hb/g faeces	0.1%
fHb 4–9.9 µg Hb/g faeces	0.6%
fHb 10–99.9 µg Hb/g faeces	3.3%
fHb 100 µg Hb/g faeces or above	20.7%

CRC, colorectal cancer.

It functions as a good 'rule-out' test but safety netting is needed to detect the occasional missed tests. The test accuracy data from Godber et al. were used by NICE to model outcomes for a hypothetical cohort of 1,000 people, assuming a prevalence of CRC of 2.2%. When a threshold of 10 µg/g faeces was applied to the cohort then the following was noted.

Correct referrals for colonoscopy (true positives): 22 cases
Incorrect referrals for colonoscopy (false positives): 229 cases
Missed CRC (false negatives): 0 cases
Colonoscopies correctly avoided (true negatives): 749 cases
Note the high false positives but zero missed CRC.

The NICE limit for a positive test that requires further assessment is therefore set at 10 µg/g faeces. In patients with suspected cancer as the FIT test is the first step in the triage of referral to secondary care.

In the UK, bowel cancer screening is offered every 2 years to men and women aged 50–74 years. People older than this can ask for a screening kit every 2 years should they so wish. A FIT test kit is sent out to the screened population with the results being provided in 2 weeks. If the test is positive, they will be called for a colonoscopy (gold standard) or CT colonogram if the former is not possible. Many polyps are picked up by this process and over time it may reduce the incidence of CRC.

Section 6: Colorectal cancer presentation and referral criteria

The presentation varies depending on the location of the cancer **(Figure 5)**.
The common symptoms are:

- Change in bowel habits such as diarrhea, constipation, or a feeling of not fully emptying the bowels lasting for a few weeks
- *Blood in or on the stool*: This can be bright red or dark, and may be intermittent.
- *Abdominal pain*: Cramping or general pain in the abdomen
- Unexplained weight loss
- Persistent fatigue which can sometimes be caused by iron deficiency anemia due to occult blood loss
- *Feeling of fullness or bloating*: A general feeling of fullness or discomfort in the abdomen
- *Lump*: A lump that can be felt in the abdomen or back passage.

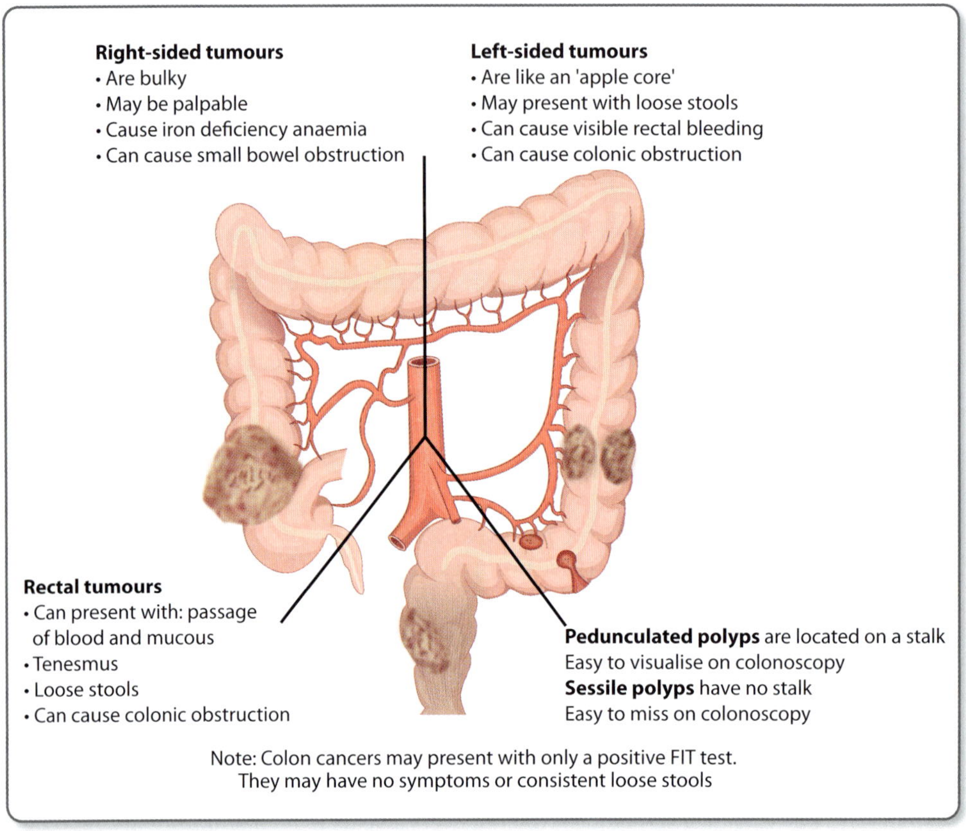

Figure 5 Presentation of colorectal malignancies.

The CRC is common worldwide with nearly 2 million detected in 2022 according to the World Cancer Research Fund (WCRF) international. China has the highest absolute numbers with over half a million new cases a year which is nearly 10 times that of the UK. India, has about 70,000 new cases a year. In terms of age standardised rates, ASR, Japan has the highest at 45.5/100,000; UK 30–40/100,000; China 25/100,000 and India 6.1/100,000 (World Cancer Research Fund).

There is some evidence to suggest that intake of vitamin C, D, and multivitamins and fish of may decrease the incidence of CRC while decreased intake of non-starchy vegetables and fruit as well as increased intake of haem may increase the risk.

Colorectal or bowel cancers arise from the columnar epithelium and are, therefore, adenocarcinomas. Anal canal cancers arise from squamous epithelium and are, therefore, squamous cell cancers; these are managed very differently from CRC.

Other cancers such as carcinoids do occur, and the principles of management are slightly different.

Criteria for a 'FAST TRACK' referral according to NICE are to offer a *FIT* test to adults presenting with:

- Abdominal mass

- Iron-deficiency anaemia
- Change in bowel habit

Aged 40 years and over with:
- Unexplained weight loss
- Abdominal pain

Aged under 50 years with rectal bleeding and any of the following unexplained symptoms or findings:
- Abdominal pain
- Weight loss

Aged 50 years and over with unexplained:
- Rectal bleeding
- Abdominal pain
- Weight loss

Aged 60 years and over with anaemia of any type:
- Changes in their bowel habit
- Positive occult blood in their faeces

Patients must be referred if they test have a FIT result of 10 μg of Hb per gram of faeces.

Patients with a rectal mass, unexplained anal mass or ulcer do not need a FIT test prior to referral.

For those whose FIT test is negative, they need referral to secondary care as a safety netting process.

Section 7: Investigations and staging

- *Digital rectal examination (DRE):* This is normally done at the time of presentation of symptoms.
- *Flexible sigmoidoscopy* for bright red rectal bleeding
- *Colonoscopy* if there is an associated change in bowel habit or a strong family history
- *CT colonogram* or CT scan if the patient is elderly or has restricted mobility
- *Positron emission tomography (PET)-CT* and *MR scans of the rectum* are other scans that are done at the request of the multidisciplinary teams

The cancers in the colon are confirmed where possible by *histological scrutiny of biopsy;* in the rectum as treatment may not always be surgical to start with histological confirmation is mandatory.

Staging of colorectal cancer

Colorectal adenocarcinoma arises in the colonic mucosa and progressively invades through the layers of bowel wall into surrounding structures, leading to peritoneal, neural, lymphatic and haematological metastasis (*Gore 1997*). This is the basis for the TNM staging and management depends on the extent of the disease as guided by TNM staging.

The TNM system is universal in its usage. The Duke's staging remains in use in common parlance.

The layers of the bowel need reiterating for the pathological clarity and understanding of the stages.

- *The mucosal layer* consists of the epithelial lining of columnar cells supported by connective tissue and a layer called muscularis *mucosa*. These together form the inner lining
- *The muscle layer* is the muscularis *propria* and the outer lining is the *serosa*.

Cuthbert Dukes, a Pathologist in London, first analysed cases of colon and rectal cancers and described a staging that is still popular because of its simplicity. It has been replaced internationally with the TNM staging (**Figure 6**) as we saw in an earlier chapter.

The Dukes' staging correlated the stage of the pathology to the duration of survival after surgery.

Dukes, described:

- *Stage A* as a cancer that is limited to the bowel
- *Stage B* as one that had invaded the wall and spread out with the bowel but not to the lymph glands
- *Stage C* as one that had spread to the lymph nodes

He did not have a stage D but simply stated it as the fourth stage when it has spread to the liver.

Note that these were observations based purely on the histology of resected specimens. *There were no radiological investigations available during his time.* The only investigative tool was the palpating hand!

He noted that the staging was related to 5-year survival. Until the establishment of screening stage A was the least commonly diagnosed but survived the longest, indicating that resection at an early stage of the disease provided greater possibility of 'cure'.

It takes a long time to collect many cases of cancer of one organ of the body such as the bowel at a general hospital admitting patients of all sorts, but this is done much more quickly in a special hospital like St. Mark's, which is intended primarily for diseases of the rectum and colon. In the last 21 years (1928–1948 inclusive) 3,220 operation specimens of intestinal cancer were examined and dissected in the laboratory of St. Mark's Hospital as follows: 2,642 cases of cancer of the rectum, 429 of the colon, 51 of the anal canal, and 98 cases of multiple malignancy.

Relation of histology to spread in rectal cancer: Cases of rectal cancer treated by radical excision have been divided into four groups according to the extent of spread of the disease as revealed by the examination of the operation specimen. In the first or initial stage the growth is limited to the bowel, the patient at this stage being described as an 'A' case. The second stage is reached when the malignant tumour has spread by direct continuity into adjoining structures, but not yet given rise to lymphatic metastases. At this stage, the patient is described as a 'B' case. The third stage is reached when the malignant growth has spread still further and given rise to lymphatic metastases. Patients at this stage are known as 'C' cases. If the malignant growth has spread to distant organs, such as the liver, this is described as the 'fourth stage'.

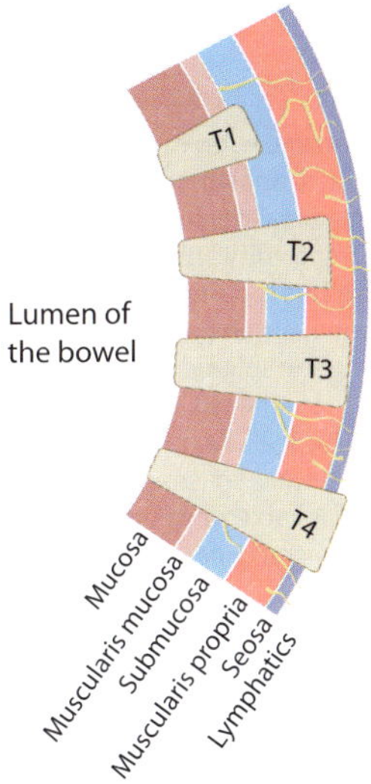

T1: Penetrates mucosa and submucosa
T2: Extends up to muscular layer – Muscularis propria
T3: Extends up to serosal layer
T4: Extends beyond serosa involves adjacent tissue/organs

N0: No nodes involved
N1: 1–3 nodes involved
N2: >4 nodes involved
M0: No metastasis detected
M1: Metastasis present

Tx, Nx, Mx: x denotes stage not assessed
Y: Prefix indicates staging has been affcted by adjuvant chemo- or radiotherapy

TME: Total mesorectal excision is the term used for rectal cancer resection
CRM: Circumferential resection margin. This must be differentiated from distal and proximal resection margins

Duke's staging remains in usage
Dukes A: Tumour extends to submucosa
Dukes B: Tumour extends through the wall
Dukes C: Tumour involves nodes
Duke did not stage metastasis

Figure 6 TNM staging of colorectal cancer.

Source: Dukes CE. The relation of histology to spread in intestinal cancer. Br J Cancer 1949; 4:59–62.

Section 8: Management of colorectal cancer

The management can be:

- A curative surgical resection when confined to the bowel wall
- A curative surgical resection after downstaging with neoadjuvant therapy. Some patients will also need postresection (adjuvant) chemotherapy
- A palliative surgical resection or stenting to improve quality of life
- Palliative chemotherapy to prolong life
- Palliative care alone for control of symptoms

Surgical management

This involves removal of the affected segment of colon along with its area of lymphatic drainage and associated blood supply (**Figure 7**).

- In the right colon cancer this would mean a *right haemicolectomy*
- Sigmoid cancers may require a *sigmoid colectomy* bearing in mind that this depends on the location. A distal sigmoid lesion will entail removal of the upper rectum and will thus be an *anterior resection* rather than a sigmoid colectomy. A proximal sigmoid lesion will entail a *left haemicolectomy* with mobilisation of the splenic flexure. True sigmoid colectomies may only be possible in a few patients with a long redundant sigmoid colon.

The blood supply of the colon dictates the safety of the resection margins. Anastomoses are carried out in areas where there is a good arterial supply

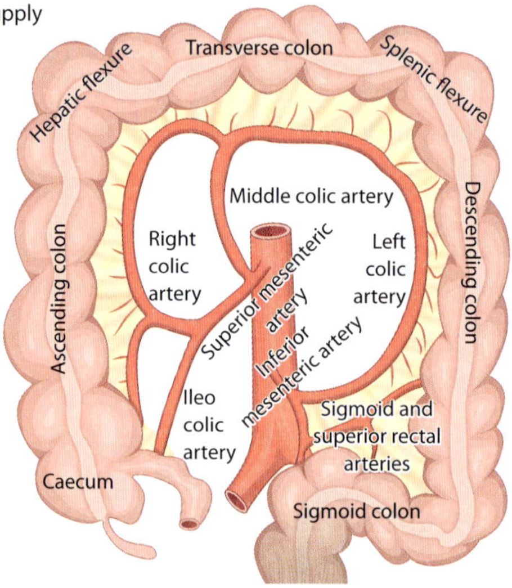

Tension and torsion must be avoided at all anastomoses as they may cause breakdown leading to leakage, morbidity and even mortality. This is particularly important in anterior resections. Mobilising the splenic flexure in these reduces the risk of anastomotic leak. At operation the newly fashioned anastomosis must be easily movable from side to side along the sacral curve

The blood supply at the splenic flexure can be variable as it depends on the arterial anastomoses between the middle and left colic arteries which occur along the arterial arcades of Drummond. Anastomosis is, therefore, best carried out either proximal to or distal to the splenic flexure

Figure 7 Impact of colonic blood supply on resections.

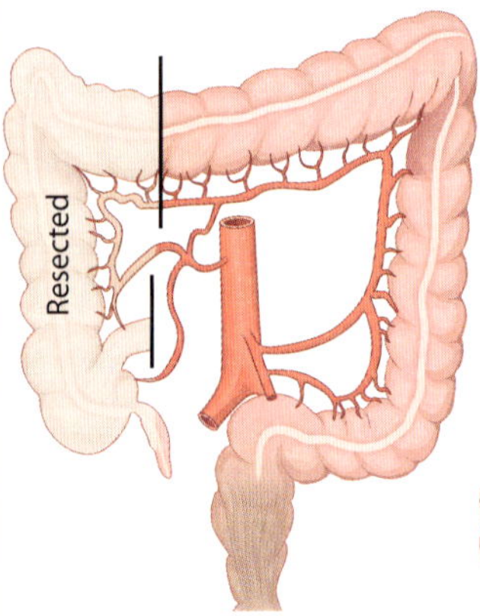

Right hemicolectomy

In a standard right hemicolectomy the **distal resection margin is proximal to the middle colic artery.** The terminal ileum, caecum, ascending colon and proximal transverse colon are resected

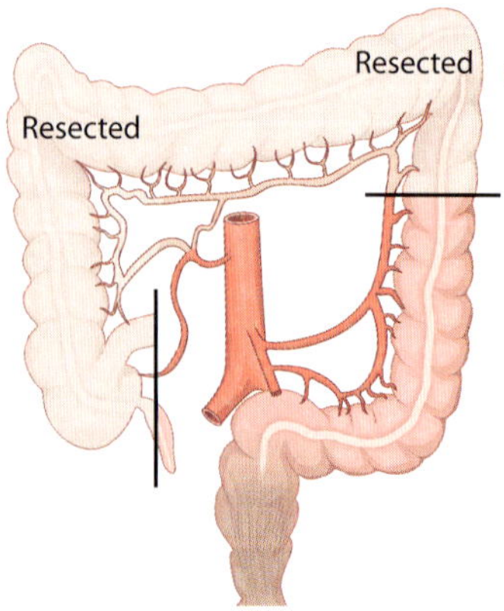

Extended right hemicolectomy

In this, the **distal resection margin is distal to the middle colic artery.** The distal resection site may lie in either the distal transverse colon or the proximal descending colon. It should never lie in the splenic flexure where the blood supply is variable

Figure 8a Colonic resections.

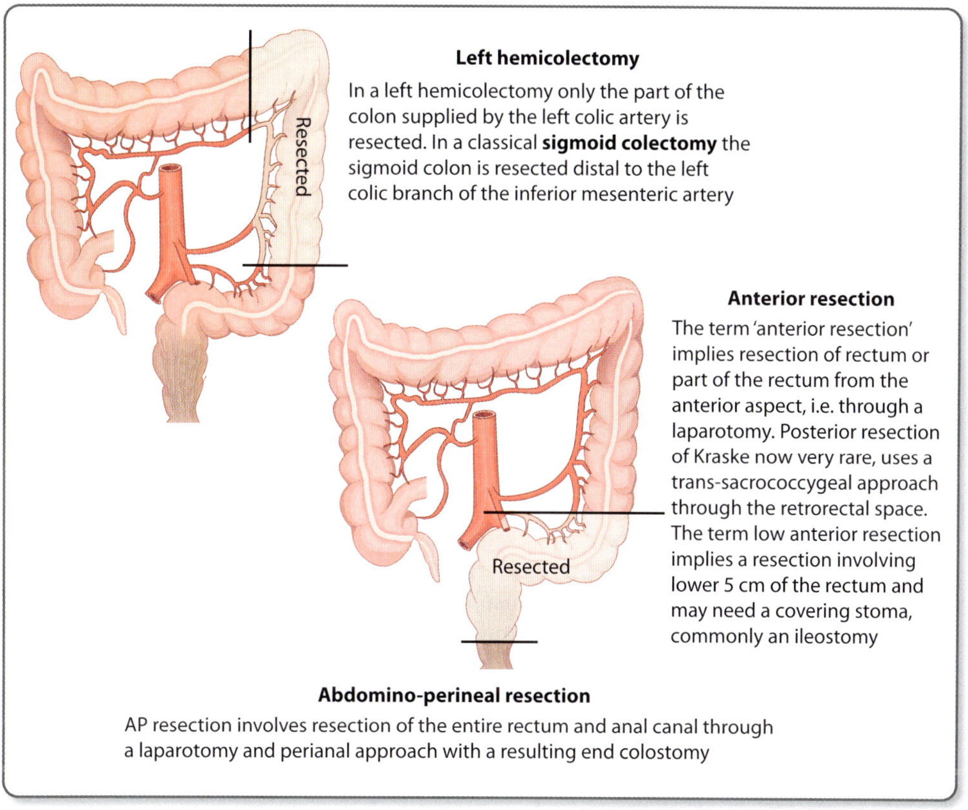

Figure 8b Colonic resections.

- Rectal cancers may be resected with a primary anastomosis called the *'anterior resection of the rectum'* with or without a covering protective ileostomy that can be reversed later
- Low-rectal cancers need resection that leaves the patient with a *colostomy* after removing the rectum by an operation called *'abdomino-perineal resection of the rectum (**Figures 8a and b**) or Hartmann's procedure'*
- *Resections can be:*
  - Open traditional laparotomy
  - Minimally invasive laparoscopic resection and external anastomosis
  - Laparoscopic resections with intracorporeal anastomosis
  - Robotic assisted operations
- Most of these operations are now done laparoscopically with gentle mobilisation and minimal blood loss aiding rapid discharge and causing less discomfort to the patient
- Enhanced recovery which includes prehabilitation is now part of the standard protocol for all elective operations
- Emergency operations will require careful evaluation and assessment of risks and benefits on an individual basis

Rectal cancers may need preoperative treatment with chemoradiotherapy to downsize the tumours. The operations for rectal cancers have undergone changes over the last few decades. The introduction of radiotherapy for select rectal cancers and advances in chemotherapy have led to a reduction in number of patients with rectal cancers needing surgery. Laparoscopic and robotic surgery has also led to more sphincter saving procedures that reduce the need for a colostomy.

An anterior resection is done 'anteriorly' as in the anatomical position, meaning that the operation is done from the abdomen without the involvement of the perineum. An *abdomino-perineal resection (APR)* of the rectum, on the other hand, requires a laparotomy as well as a perineal dissection. This was pioneered by *Miles.* It is carried out for low rectal tumours that do not have sufficient distal clearance to permit a primary anastomosis. Inevitably it requires a colostomy.

A *Hartmann's operation* does not require a perineal dissection. It removes most of the rectum without a rejoining anastomosis. The distal end is closed and the proximal end is brought out as a colostomy.

Role of chemotherapy and radiotherapy

These are discussed for each patient at the *multidisciplinary team meeting.* In colonic cancers, the role of chemotherapy, prior to surgery is to downstage the disease to enable a curative resection. Prior to the decision to use neoadjuvant chemotherapy, the total extent of the disease must be clearly defined and the disease must be histologically confirmed. The definition of the extent of the disease requires radiological assistance in the form of a CT TAP – *T*horax, *A*bdomen, *P*elvis. A PET-CT may be needed to ensure the absence of metastatic disease.

Section 9: Complications of colorectal cancers

These may present acutely due to:

- Local invasion
- Metastatic spread

Local invasion is due to tumour growth and may lead to:

- Obstruction
- Perforation
- Haemorrhage
- Fistula formation

These can be managed surgically in fit patients.

In colonic obstruction due to left-sided malignancies of the colon, the area of tenderness may be located over the caecum. Caecum is the thinnest part of the colon that has the maximal diameter. In colonic obstruction in the distal or left colon, the wall of the caecum being thinner tends to distend early and more than the rest of the colon. (Laplace stated that the pressure on the wall is greatest where the radius is largest – caecum being the widest and thinnest is the easiest to distend with increasing pressure). Progressive distension causes ischaemia due to stretching and may lead to caecal perforation. This distension is maximal if the ileo-caecal valve is competent. When the valve is incompetent, the presentation may involve small bowel obstruction.

On radiological imaging, if the caecum is distended beyond 12 cm, it should raise suspicion of impending ischaemia or caecal perforation. In cases of bowel obstruction, it is good to follow the 3:6:9:12 rule. If small bowel is distended above, 3 cm, the colon above 6 cm and caecum above 9 cm, obstruction should be suspected. If caecum is greater than 12 cm risk of perforation increases.

The management in these situations is dependent upon, as always, the suitability of the patient for surgery.

If the patient is suitable for surgery – the extent of the disease is assessed with an immediate CT scan.

If curative resection is feasible, then it should be undertaken. If palliative treatment is needed, then stenting can be carried out to improve the quality of residual life. Surgical intervention can be carried out with resection and restoration of continuity or diversion with a colostomy or ileostomy depending on the location of the tumour. In left-sided and transverse colonic tumours, stenting may be possible for symptomatic relief. In very selected patients, it may be used as a bridge to delayed resection and restorative surgery. There are some concerns regarding the oncological safety of stenting as a bridge to definitive surgery as some studies suggest that it may increase local and peritoneal recurrence.

Caecal or ascending colon cancers can cause small bowel obstruction. They may be amenable to immediate resection and primary anastomosis.

Palliative stoma may also be an option for consideration in some patients.

Metastatic complications

Management of metastases depends on:

- *Number:* Solitary or multiple
- *Isolation:* Single organ or more
- Extent of local disease and presence of systemic spread
- Performance score of the patient
- Comorbidities
- Delivering better quality of life
- Prolonging survival

Liver metastases may be detected synchronously, 15% (initial investigations) or metachronously 15% (during follow-up). They may be asymptomatic or present with jaundice, hepatomegaly, and right upper quadrant pain.

Factors influencing treatment choice:

- Type of cancer
- Extent of disease
- Patient's overall health
- Patient's preferences

The options for treatment are:

- Surgical resection
- Locoregional therapy
- Chemotherapy
- Targeted therapy
- Immunotherapy
- Palliative care

Hepatic resection is the gold standard of treatment of colorectal liver metastatic (CLRM) disease. Surgery to remove cancerous tissue is the primary treatment option if the metastases are limited and resectable. In some cases, surgery offers the best chance for a cure. Liver resection, however, is a major procedure, and not all patients are suitable candidates. Selection of patients for resection depends upon *anatomic factors*:

- Ability to obtain a R0 resection
- Tumour relationship to major vessels and bile ducts
- Future liver remnant (FLR) volume

When metastatic disease that is located primarily in the liver is noted, it must be discussed the hepatobiliary team as to the suitability of hepatic resection, alternative treatments or systemic chemotherapy. Discussions need to be had regarding the *sequence of the treatment* in synchronous lesions. The *primary first, liver first* or *simultaneous* approach needs careful consideration based on the logistics. There was no difference in the outcome between these two approaches. The resection of the metastatic deposit may be carried out prior to colorectal surgery, synchronously or postcolonic resection.

Locoregional therapies

These therapies focus on liver metastases by destroying them or blocking their blood supply.

- *Ablation:* Uses heat or cold to destroy cancer cells.
- *Radioembolisation:* Delivers radioactive particles to liver tumours
- *Stereotactic body radiation therapy (SBRT):* Applies precise high-dose radiation to tumours.
- *Selective internal radiotherapy (SIRT)*: Delivers radioactive beads to the metastatic deposit through the branches of the hepatic artery the causing damage to the cancer cells and their blood supply while minimising harm to normal cells. SBRT by contrast is a type of external beam radiation therapy that targets the tumour from multiple angles with precise radiation beams.
- Histotripsy is a new technology that focuses high energy ultrasound on metastatic deposits to destroy the cancer cells

Locoregional therapies can shrink tumours, manage symptoms, or prepare for delayed surgery.

Chemotherapy

- Chemotherapy is employed to shrink tumours
- Control the spread of cancer
- Improve survival rates, especially when the cancer has disseminated beyond the liver

Chemotherapy drugs can be administered intravenously or directly into the liver via a catheter.

Chemoembolisation blocks the blood flow to the tumour.

Targeted therapies

These medications are designed to target specific molecules or pathways that contribute to the growth and spread of cancer. Examples of targeted therapies used in the treatment of liver cancer include sorafenib, lenvatinib, and regorafenib.

Immunotherapy

Immunotherapy utilises the body's own immune system to combat cancer.

Genomic factors such as *RAS* mutations are detrimental to overall and disease-free survival.

Clinical risk score (CRS), otherwise known as the 'Fong CRS' is frequently used after retrospectively reviewing 1,001 hepatectomies for colorectal liver metastasis (CRLM) at a single institution. The authors identified five factors that were associated with long-term outcomes:

1. Node-positive primary
2. Disease-free interval (DFI) from primary to metastasis diagnosis < 12 months
3. Number of tumours > 1
4. Largest hepatic tumour diameter > 5 cm
5. Carcinoembryonic antigen (CEA) > 200 ng/mL

Each factor was assigned a point value of 1, with increasing scores portending a worse disease-free survival.

Alternative treatments need consideration and discussion when hepatic resection is not feasible.

The metastatic liver disease can also be downstaged with chemotherapy prior to resection. In all these complicated cases, discussions with the multidisciplinary team are most beneficial.

Disappearing liver metastases

These are lesions present on initial imaging that disappear after chemotherapy demonstrating a complete response. These are challenging to manage and benefit from follow-up.

Role of intraoperative ultrasound (IOUS) imaging: In many patients with hepatic metastases, an intraoperative assessment after liver mobilisation, IOUS is employed to assess the liver for lesions. Ferrero et al. retrospectively identified patients with disappearing liver metastasis using IOUS. The median size of the lesions detected on IOUS was 6 mm. Moderate-to-severe hepatic steatosis ($p = 0.016$) was the reason that these could not be detected by imaging.

Lung metastases may be solitary and isolated to the lung alone or be part of a systemic manifestation of the disease.

Systemic manifestations require systemic therapy.

Various options are feasible for *localised disease.*

- Local resection
- Radiotherapy
- *Stereotactic body radiation therapy:* This is focussed and high-dose radiotherapy. Can be ablative in higher fractionated doses.

Peritoneal carcinomatosis with ascites can be managed by 'paracentesis for symptomatic' relief of ascites.

Hyperthermic intraperitoneal chemotherapy (HIPEC): It can be used in selected patients with limited peritoneal disease.

Complications of surgery

Systemic complications such as cardiopulmonary complications and wound infections sometimes leading to dehiscence may occur.

The most dreaded complication is an *anastomotic leak*. This is more common in left-sided and rectal resections, especially low-rectal resections. In low-rectal resections leak rates are higher when resection follows chemoradiotherapy. This typically occurs 4–8 days after surgery. Early recognition, introduction of *sepsis six protocol* and immediate surgery with resection of the anastomosis and formation of a stoma are key to reduction in morbidity and mortality. In a very select few a primary re-anastomosis may be feasible. These patients are best managed in a critical care setting postoperatively.

Section 10: Follow-up

The NICE recommendation following curative resection for detection of local recurrence and distant metastasis is for regular *CEA* and *CT scan* of the thorax, abdomen and pelvis annually for the first 3 years.

Colonoscopy is recommended at the end of the first year and at the third year. Subsequent follow-up can be scheduled after mutual discussions.

Role of carcinoembryonic antigen

*C*arcino-*E*mbryonic *A*ntigen is found in embryos in the endodermal epithelium. It disappears after birth but small quantities remain in the colon. This antigen is a useful marker in the period following treatment of CRC. It is non-specific and has a low sensitivity for colon cancers (more false positives). Elevated levels can be found in colon, breast, liver and lung cancers.

The specificity rises with the occurrence of recurrence following treatment.

The lack of sensitivity means it is not an ideal tool for screening.

A base line value prior to initiating treatment will assist as a guide to the completeness of resection and the occurrence of recurrence in the follow-up period.

The recommendation is for CEA levels to be monitored 3 monthly for the first 2 years after resection along with annual CT scans and subsequently at 6-monthly intervals for 5 years. This recommendation may vary in different countries.

Serum carcinoembryonic antigen levels of significance

- Healthy, non-smoking adults ≤3.0 μg/L
- In smokers, normal limits <5 μg/L
- Pretreatment serum CEA levels > 5 μg/L but <10 μg/L suggests localised disease and a low likelihood of recurrence, hence a *favourable prognosis.*
- A serum level of >10 μg/L indicates a higher likelihood of recurrence and poor prognosis.
- Serum titres of >20 μg/L are usually associated with metastatic disease in colon cancers (and breast cancers).
- For CRC, a CEA threshold of 2.5 μg/L carries a sensitivity of 82% and a specificity of 80%, while a threshold of 10 μg/L carries a sensitivity of 68% and specificity of 97%

In addition, the Cochrane review (2015) shows that a rise in CEA does not occur in up to 20% of patients with a true recurrence (false negatives). The current evidence supports using the highest cut-off point assessed (10 µg/L) to detect recurrence, but that *adding another diagnostic modality* (e.g. a single scan of the chest, abdomen and pelvis at 12–18 months) is necessary in order to avoid the missed cases.

Section 11: Survival in colorectal cancer (Tables 5 and 6)

Table 5 Survival after colorectal cancer.

Duke stage	Percentage detected	5-year survival rate
A	15%	94%
B	35%	87%
C	50%	58%
RJ Heald		

Table 6 SEER survival.

SEER stage	5 year relative survival rate
Localised	91%
Regional	73%
Distant	13%
All stages combined	63%

Section 12: Anal canal cancer

Anal cancers are not very common. They constitute up to 3–4% of anorectal cancers. They can be:

- Squamous cell cancer of anal canal (SCCA) – the most common
- Adenocarcinoma from the anal glands – rare
- Melanoma
- Basal cell cancer

The most common type of anal cancer is a squamous cell cancer.

Typically, these cancers are located at and below the dentate line. The cancers may occur in the anal canal or in the anal margin (more common). The anal margin is the area of hair bearing skin for a radius of 5 cm around the external opening of the anal canal.

Anal margin and perianal cancers are treated as SCC elsewhere in the body.

The morphology of these is that of moderately well-differentiated keratinising squamous cell cancer (SCC). The lymphatic drainage of anal margin cancers is not to the intraperitoneal nodes but to the groin and to the external and common iliac nodes in the retroperitoneum.

Risk factors:

- Anal SCC cancers are related to HPV-16 and -18
- They occur in patients with HIV as HPV infections may coexist

- Insertive intercourse with multiple partners
- Smoking

The presentation is similar to rectal cancers. There is often a delay with mistaken diagnosis of haemorrhoids. Commonly they present with:

- Bleeding
- Lump
- Ulcers
- Pruritus

Clinical examination must include a digital rectal examination and proctoscopy. Needless to say, the examination of the abdomen must be accompanied by an examination of the groin nodes.

Investigations are similar to CRC and involves the use of colonoscopy, CT scans and MRI.

TNM staging is used for staging and is based on the size of the primary lesion and the presence of nodal or adjacent organ involvement. Metastasis can occur to the liver and lungs.

Treatment is normally dictated by the TNM staging. The prognosis is mostly good.

Treatment modalities

- *Surgery* – with local resection or abdomino perineal resection in a few cases. Groin node clearance in a select number
- *Radiotherapy*
- *Chemotherapy* with 5-fluorouracil and the like
- *Immunotherapy*

Chemoradiotherapy for squamous cell cancer of the anal canal

In 1974, Norman Nigro developed a 'first step' therapy for invasive anal carcinoma to help to shrink tumours before surgery. The standard method of treatment for SCC of the anal canal was APR. In trying to downsize larger tumours prior to surgery, Dr Nigro and colleagues noted complete tumour regression in some patients using their protocol of treatment with fluorouracil (5-FU)-based chemotherapy administered concurrently with radiation and the addition of either mitomycin or porfiromycin chemotherapy. This study made possible the cure anal carcinoma without surgery and the need for an end colostomy.

The study was on 104 patients and he demonstrated complete clinical and pathologic response in most. The 'Nigro protocol' has now reduced the need for APR to those with residual or recurrent disease.

Section 13: The key points of rectal bleeding

Points of note: Management of rectal bleeding

- Haemorrhoidal bleeding is normally bright red and painless
- Blood may be noted on paper, on wiping or in the pan
- Blood in the pan can appear to be a lot more than the actual amount due to dilution
- Blood in the paper could be due to fissure as well as haemorrhoids, polyps or low rectal or anal cancer

- Mucous and blood is common with inflammatory disease
- Constipation is a precursor in many cases of fissure and haemorrhoids but not always
- Diverticular bleed can be profuse
- Malignant tumours and polyps may cause bleeding in isolation or mixed with mucous
- Polyps or cancers of the rectum can present as haemorrhoids
- Painful bleeding is often associated with fissure in ano
- Typically, painful rectal bleeding where the pain lasts after voiding is consistent with a fissure in ano
- In patients with a fissure in ano, the patient may volunteer the information that voiding stools is like passing glass!
- The fissure may be visible on inspection, often being located just at the anal verge at 6 or 12 o'clock positions
- Most fissures are located posteriorly
- Anterior fissures are more common in women
- In haemorrhoidal bleeding the stools are typically separate from the blood
- Thrombosed haemorrhoids or a *perianal haematoma* can present acutely with a painful lump
- Perianal haematoma presents with acute pain that is followed by a lump in the perineum. The lump is due to a bleed into an external skin tag or into the skin. It swells and becomes painful due to the pressure that builds in the contained space
- Release of tension by opening the haematoma resolves the pain; if, on the other hand, a non-operative approach is followed, the relief occurs with resorption of the haematoma that normally takes place in about 5 days; this is thus referred to as the *'5-day painful condition'*
- *A digital rectal examination is mandatory.* This may not be possible in patients with fissure in ano as the acute condition is very painful
- Where there is doubt an examination under anaesthesia is needed urgently to exclude other causes such as a painful malignancy
- *Proctoscopy* is needed in all patients presenting with a clear history of bright red rectal bleeding that is separate from stools; a digital rectal examination is likely to *define the cause.* Proctoscopy will in most *cases define the site* of the haemorrhoids and assist in planning further treatment
- *Sigmoidoscopy* or colonoscopy is needed to confirm the diagnosis and exclude other causes
- *Colonoscopy* may be needed if the cause of the rectal bleeding is not obvious. This is likely to be the case, when the patient is older and offers a family history of bowel cancer. It may also be indicated when the type of bleeding is thought not to be related to anorectal pathology based on the history
- As always, a good history is important in elucidating the cause of the presentation
- Lifestyle changes will need discussions with the patient including avoidance of constipation where haemorrhoids are present
- *FIT* (faecal immunochemical test) is clearly not necessary when the bleeding is obvious. The indication for it is more in patients with recent change in bowel habit when there is a need to exclude neoplastic lesions
- *Faecal calprotectin* is a marker of inflammation of the bowel. This may be needed in patients who present with rectal bleeding associated with change in bowel habit.

Section 14: Appendix – key papers

1. *Total mesorectal excision (TME) of rectum:* In a historic, innovative and paradigm-shifting manuscript published in 1982 in the *British Journal of Surgery*, Professor R. J. (Bill) Heald described the importance of the mesorectum in rectal cancer. The *TME* was first described 40 years ago by *Richard Heald.* The purpose of this article is to point out importance of this surgical procedure. Starting from first attempts to surgically cure rectal carcinoma in the nineteenth century through *Miles'* operation at the beginning of the 20th century results were not satisfactory due to high number of local recurrences after resections for rectal cancer. Progress in surgical technique and knowledge of anatomy and embryology of the rectum led to development of TME.

   Principle of TME is surprisingly simple: removal of the rectum with complete embryonic space containing lymph nodes which are site of primary dissemination of the disease (**Figure 9**).
2. *A key paper on this was published by RJ Heald and RD Ryall in the Lancet [1986; 1(8496):1479–1482].* This paper showed that when complete resection of the mesorectum was combined with resection for low- and mid-rectal adenocarcinoma, there was not only a low recurrence rate but also longer survival. TME was promoted by Heald for adenocarcinoma with the distal edge ≤ 15 cm from the anal verge, undergoing a curative resection. This was a single centre and single surgeon study with

TME: Total mesorectal excision is complete sharp excision of visceral mesorectum to the level of the levator, with the preservation of the pelvic nerves. It is the gold standard for the treatment of rectal cancers

Defects in the mesorectum fascia on a tissue sample are associated with pelvic recurrence. Positive circumferential resection margin **(CRM)** had a 78% local recurrence, compared to 10% if edges were negative. For patients with positive edges, 40% developed distant metastases, compared to 12% of those with negative edges

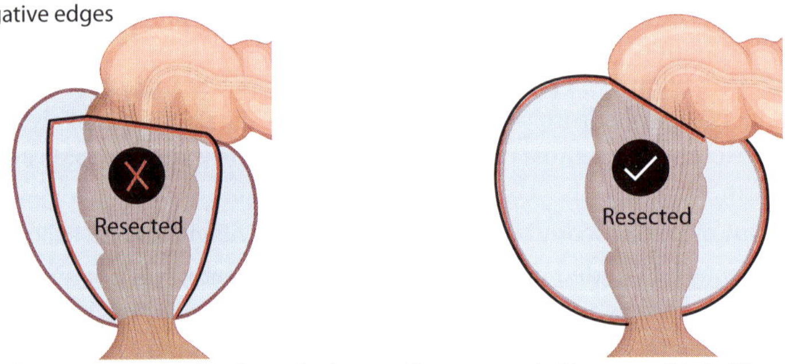

- Mesorectal nodes are tiny measuring 3 mm in size
- 54% of the nodes are located posteriorly
- 92% of the nodes are located in the upper half of the upper two-thirds of the rectum
- Intramural distal spread of rectal cancer is rare
- Extramural spread occurs proximally and distally
- TME clears nodes of the upper two-thirds of the rectum but lateral pelvic spread may occur in the lower third compromising clearance

For tumours in the upper third of the rectum a **'Partial mesorectum excision'** may be performed. In this case, the mesorectum dissection is performed 5 cm distal from the lower edge of the tumour, in a plane of 90% on the rectal wall, with a sharp mesorectum dissection

Figure 9 Laparoscopic resection of rectal cancers.

lack of comparison. In this study, the corrected cumulative probability of tumour free 5-year survival by Duke staging was as follows:

- Duke stage A 94%
- Duke stage B 87%
- Duke stage C 58%

Operative mortality was 2.6% for a study population of 115 undergoing curative restorative proctocolectomy.

In the UK, this study altered the management of low- and mid-rectal cancers. Laparoscopic resection subsequently improved the access for resection and improved overall survival compared to the previous 'smash and grab' approach of excision of the mesorectum.

3. *Long and short course radiotherapy and timing of surgery:* Radiotherapy reduces the risk of local recurrence after rectal cancer resection. In 1997, the Swedish Rectal Cancer Trial was the first RCT to demonstrate a clear benefit of neoadjuvant RT compared to surgery alone. There was debate about short and long course radiotherapy and the timing of surgery.

   The Stockholm III trial was a multicentre RCT. From October 1998 to January 2013, 840 patients were recruited and randomised; 385 patients in the three-arm randomisation, of whom 129 patients were randomly assigned to short-course radiotherapy, 128 to short-course radiotherapy with delay, and 128 to long-course radiotherapy with delay, and 455 patients in the two-arm randomisation, of whom 228 were randomly assigned to short-course radiotherapy and 227 to short-course radiotherapy with delay. Long-course radiotherapy with delay is similar to both short-course radiotherapy regimens, but *prolongs the treatment time* substantially. The study compared long-course RT with the standard expected delay for surgical treatment (4–8 weeks), short-course RT without delay, and short-course RT with delay. They observed no difference in the incidence of local recurrence, distant metastasis or overall survival among the three groups. They did, however, demonstrate *significantly fewer postoperative complications in the groups that had delayed surgical treatment.* Most importantly, the study re-emphasised that either short- or long-course RT with concurrent administration of chemotherapy was integral to reducing local recurrence.

4. *Habr-Gama A, Perez RO, Nadalin W, et al. Operative versus nonoperative treatment for stage 0 distal rectal cancer following chemoradiation therapy: long-term results. Annals of Surgery. 2004; 240:711–717.*

   Operative versus non-operative management of rectal cancer: Management of rectal cancers have become more complex with the finding that long course radiotherapy that was used to downstage tumours had indeed caused complete regression with delay to interventional surgery. Surgical intervention has consequences of colostomy and other complications, as does radiotherapy. In a select group of patients, however, surgery could be avoided or deferred with close follow-up with radiological imaging and CEA.

   A seminal paper by Angelita Habr Gama reported in 2004, has changed the way rectal cancers are managed. Two-hundred sixty-five patients with distal rectal adenocarcinoma considered resectable were treated by neoadjuvant chemoradiation (CRT) with 5-FU, leucovorin and 5040 cGy. Patients with incomplete clinical response were referred to radical surgical resection. Patients with incomplete clinical response treated by surgery resulting in stage p0 were compared to patients with complete clinical response treated by non-operative treatment. Statistical analysis was performed using $\chi 2$, Student t-test and Kaplan–Meier curves.

Overall and disease-free 10-year survival rates were 97.7 and 84%.

Observation group: 71 patients (26.8%) complete clinical response following CRT (observation group).

Resection group: Twenty-two patients (8.3%) showed incomplete clinical response and pT0N0M0 resected specimens. In the Resection group, nine definitive colostomies and seven diverting temporary ileostomies were performed. Two patients in the Resection group died of the disease.

There were three systemic recurrences in each group.

There were two endorectal recurrences in 'Observation Group'. 5-year overall and disease-free survival rates were:

- *Resection group:* 88 and 83%, respectively
- *Observation group:* 100 and 92%, respectively

First-line chemoradiotherapy for distal rectal adenocarcinoma can result in complete clinical and pathological response in a proportion of patients. In these patients, surgical resection may not offer a survival benefit. It may be associated with temporary or definitive stoma, morbidity and mortality.

5. *ELAPE. Simon W, Raymond Y, Shehara M, et al. Surgical Techniques for Abdominoperineal Resection for Rectal Cancer: One Size Does Not Fit All. Front Surg 2022; 9.*

   Abdominoperineal resection *(APR)* of rectal cancer is associated with poorer oncological outcomes than anterior resection. This may be due to higher rates of *intraoperative perforation (IOP)* and *circumferential resection margin (CRM)* involvement causing higher recurrence rates and surgical complications. To address these concerns, several centres advocated a change in technique from a standard APR to *a more radical extra-levator abdominoperineal excision (ELAPE).* Initial reports showed that ELAPE reduced IOP rates and CRM involvement but increased wound complications and surgical duration. However, many of these studies had unacceptable rates of IOP and CRM involvement before retraining in ELAPE. This may indicate that it was a suboptimal surgical technique, which improved upon training, that had influenced the high CRM and IOP rates rather than the technique itself. Subsequent studies demonstrated that the CRM involvement rate for ELAPE was not always lower than for standard APR and, in some cases, significantly higher. The morbidity of ELAPE can be high, with studies reporting higher adverse events than APR, especially in terms of wound complications from the larger perineal incision required in ELAPE. Whether ELAPE improves short- or long-term oncological outcomes for patients has not been clearly demonstrated. The authors propose that all centres performing rectal cancer surgery audit surgical outcomes of patients undergoing APR or ELAPE and examine CRM involvement, IOP rates, and local recurrence rates, preferably through a national body. If rates of adverse technical or oncological outcomes exceed acceptable levels, then retraining in the appropriate surgical techniques may be indicated.

6. *Delaney CP, Fazio VW, Senagore AJ, et al. 'Fast track' postoperative management protocol for patients with high comorbidity undergoing complex abdominal and pelvic colorectal surgery.* Br J Surg 2001; 88:1533–1538.

This article demonstrated that enhanced recovery protocols could be applied to patients undergoing complex abdominal surgery. Those with comorbidities stayed a day longer. Overall, the group had a shorter length of stay without incurring harm. The readmission rates were also low.

7. *Ljungqvist O, Scott M, Fearon KC. Enhanced Recovery After Surgery: A Review. JAMA Surg 2017; 152:292–298.*

   Enhanced recovery after surgery (ERAS) is a multimodal, multidisciplinary approach applied initially to the care of CRC surgery patients. It involves a team led by a co-ordinator including surgeons, anaesthetists and staff from units that care for the surgical patient. The care protocol is based on published evidence. It has been shown to decrease stress of the operation. The ERAS Society publishes updated guidelines for many operations regarding:

   - *Carbohydrate drinks 2 hours before surgery* (This seeks to retain the anabolic state prior to surgery instead of starvation that pushes the patient to a catabolic state at the onset of surgery taking them further down the pathway of the metabolic response to surgery).
   - *Minimally invasive approaches* instead of large incisions
   - Management of fluids to seek balance rather than large volumes of intravenous fluids
   - Avoidance of or *early removal of drains* and tubes
   - *Early mobilisation*
   - Serving of drinks and food the day of the operation (This is possibly useful in selected patients and must be used with judgement.)

   'Enhanced recovery after surgery' protocols have resulted in shorter length of hospital and may contribute to reduction in complications and readmissions.

Conclusion

Multidisciplinary management of colorectal cancer has driven tailored treatment. In rectal cancer, neoadjuvant treatment and total mesorectal excision, have improved outcomes. Advances in minimally invasive techniques, particularly laparoscopic and robotic surgery, have enhanced surgical precision, reduced perioperative morbidity, and facilitated faster recovery. When combined with Enhanced Recovery After Surgery (ERAS) protocols, these innovations have shortened hospital stay and improved postoperative outcomes without compromising oncologic safety.

Chapter 8

Thyroid disease

Srinivasan Ravi

Section 1: Gross anatomy

Refer to **Figure 1**

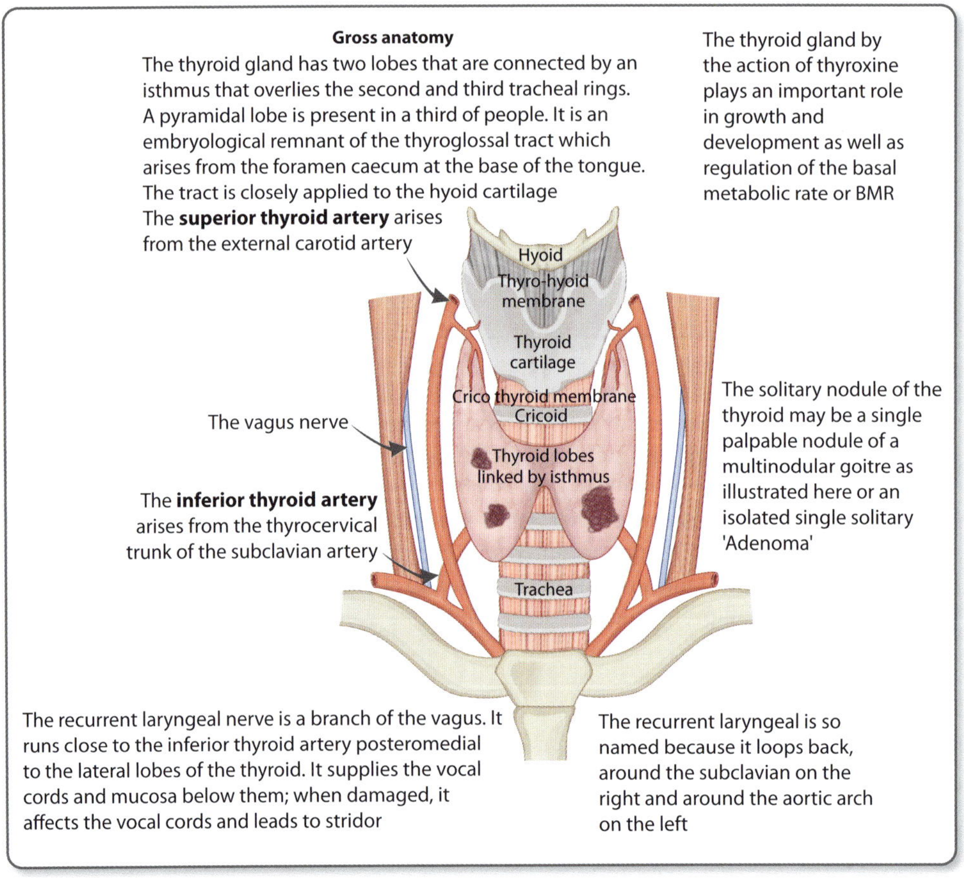

Figure 1 The anatomy of the thyroid gland.

Section 2: Physiology and investigations

The production of thyroxine by the thyroid gland from the inorganic iodine in food is a multistep-regulated process. The uptake of iodine by the thyroid gland is determined by its availability in the circulating blood and is a key step in the formation of thyroxine. The ability of the thyroid gland to concentrate iodine is the basis for many clinical investigations and its understanding is paramount to the management of thyroid diseases such as hypothyroidism, hyperthyroidism, and malignancies such as papillary and follicular carcinoma.

Histophysiology

The gland contains numerous follicles with capillaries between follicles. Each of these follicles has a single layer of follicular cells that surround the lumen or cavity. The lumen contains the colloid which is the storehouse of thyroglobulin. Thyroglobulin is synthesised by follicular cells and secreted into the lumen to help to synthesise thyroxine.

Step 1: Absorption of inorganic iodine

Inorganic iodine from food is taken up by the thyroid gland and converted to organic iodine as the first step in the synthesis of thyroxine. *Thyroid peroxidase (TPO)* mediates the oxidation and organification of iodine following its uptake.

$$\text{Inorganic iodine} \xrightarrow{\text{TPO}} \text{Organic iodine}$$

Step 2: Combination of organic iodine with tyrosine

Organic iodine is combined with tyrosine to make monoiodotyrosine or MIT. Two molecules of MIT combine to form di-iodotyrosine or DIT. MIT + DIT = T3. T4 is likewise (DIT + DIT) formed by further addition of iodine. This is then retained in the thyroid gland as thyroglobulin which is a mixture of T4 and T3 in the ratio of 11:1. T3 formation also occurs in the peripheral tissues other than the thyroid. *T3 is the active moiety.*

Step 3: Thyroxine release by thyroid-stimulating hormone

The release of thyroxine is controlled by thyroid-stimulating hormone (TSH). TSH is released from the pituitary in a classical negative feedback system. Thyrotrophin-releasing hormone (TRH) arising from the hypothalamus in turn controls TSH.

*Feedback mechanism (**Figure 2**) regulates the release of thyroxine:* Increased T4 acts on hypothalamus and pituitary gland to decrease TSH and vice versa. *TSH is thus the controller of the activity of the thyroid gland* and its regulation plays a major role in management of thyroid disease.

When the thyroxine in blood stream is low, it leads to more release of thyrotrophin, TSH. This leads to stimulation of the thyroid cells to increase thyroxine production.

When there is more thyroxine in bloodstream, it leads to lessen TSH activity and to reduced thyroxine release from the thyroid gland.

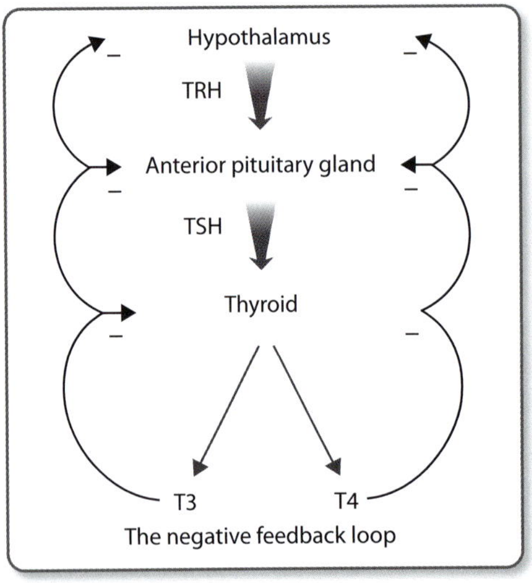

Figure 2 The feedback mechanism.

TSH is thus a primary regulator of thyroid function.

Lack of availability of iodine has a similar effect as it leads to less thyroxine production leading to more TSH causing hyperplasia and hypertrophy of thyroid cells leading to goitre.

Iodine is mostly found in the oceans of the world. It vaporises as part of the water cycle falling as rain. Most iodine in food is derived from the soil. The cycling of iodine may be incomplete leaving many areas of the world lacking in iodine, needing supplementation in diet as iodised salt. It is found in sea food and as an additive in bread.

Iodine deficiency is well-recognised in mountainous regions of the world including the *Alpine areas of Europe, the Himalayas* in the Indian Subcontinent, and mountain ranges of China, and South America.

Iodine deficiency in the diet leads to *goitre,* referred to as *Struma* because of its early recognition along the Struma River that flows between Bulgaria and Greece.

Iodine deficiency in mothers leads to foetal deficiency that manifests as *cretinism* with short stature, spasticity, and deaf mutism. It is a recognised cause of infant mortality and neurocognitive disorders in infants. *Iodine and thyroxine are an important factor in the development of the brain.* Supplementing diet with iodine has reduced the disorders of iodine deficiency.

Actions of thyroxine T4

- *Regulation of metabolic rate* by increasing oxygen consumption and heat production (calorigenic)
- *Regulation of growth and development:* Well-known effect on brain function – cretinism
- Synergistically with growth hormone and influences *differentiation and growth of tissue*
- *Enhances actions of catecholamines* by affecting excitability

Thyroid function tests

The commonly used tests to assess the function of the thyroid gland are the levels of:

- Thyroid-stimulating hormone
- T4
- T3
- Thyroid autoantibodies – Thyroid peroxidase antibodies (TPO), elevated in Hashimoto's disease; thyroglobulin antibodies elevated in auto immune thyroiditis and thyroid stimulating immunoglobulins, elevated in Grave's disease.

Section 3: Solitary and multinodular goitre

Enlargement of the thyroid gland secondary to deficiency of iodine is commonly called a goitre. The deficiency of iodine could be *dietary* or due to *physiological stress* such as pregnancy, menopause, leading to a *colloid goitre.*

Typically, in an iodine-deficient goitre the whole of the thyroid is *uniformly enlarged* and the *thyroid function is likely to remain normal.* In most situations, a non-interventional medical management will suffice. This is dependent on the thyroid status. It may require, replacement thyroxine, iodine or in the case of an overactive thyroid, anti-thyroid medication. Surgical intervention is necessary only for cosmesis or pressure effects.

Diffuse enlargement of the whole gland is seen in Colloid goitre, Grave's disease and Hashimoto's disease.

Solitary nodule

Solitary nodule could be a *single palpable nodule* of a multinodular goitre, an adenoma, or rarely a carcinoma.

Thyroid disease can present as generalised enlargement of the whole gland or enlargements in nodules – solitary or multinodular.

The work-up of a solitary nodule includes the following:

- Assessment of the clinical status of thyroid
- Assessment of the biochemical status of thyroid
- Assessment of thyroid autoantibodies to rule out Hashimoto's or other forms of autoimmune disease
- Ultrasound examination of thyroid determines if the nodule is:
  - Cystic or solid
  - Multiple or single
- Fine needle cytology – to exclude papillary cancers. The cytology cannot differentiate between follicular adenoma and follicular carcinoma.

The distinction between a follicular adenoma and a carcinoma is based on histological evidence of a breach in the capsule and presence of tumour emboli in the vessels. Neither of these changes can be seen on cytology.

In certain situations, an isotope scan of the thyroid gland may be needed for diagnostic purposes and this is usually performed using radioisotope – Technetium-99m or I^{131}.

The scan may show an increased or decreased take up in a nodule of the gland. When the uptake is higher than the surrounding gland it lights up as a bright spot and is referred to as a *hot nodule*. Hot nodules are almost always benign and signify an autonomous nodule that is producing an excess of thyroxine. These patients tend to have a *hyperthyroid* state.

When the uptake is less than that of the rest of the gland it is referred to as a *cold nodule. Only about 15% of cold nodules are malignant.*

Solitary adenoma – management

When an isolated single nodule is detected, it is deemed a solitary adenoma. Most of these are well-encapsulated follicular adenomas and can be observed without surgical intervention in most cases. When there is doubt about a carcinoma surgical intervention is needed. Surgical treatment depends on the diagnosis.

The indication for surgery is the three Cs:

1. Cosmesis, if it progressively becomes large
2. Compression
3. Cancer

Compression is manifest by:

- Difficulty in swallowing
- Difficulty in breathing
- Hoarseness of voice

This history must be obtained. *Hoarseness of voice* is indicative of malignancy and involves pressure on the recurrent laryngeal nerve. *Voice fatigue,* (inability to speak loudly at the end of a day or to sing high notes), occurs in some patients with a large goitre due to traction on the external laryngeal nerve. In those situations which are now rare in the west, the goitre becomes very large and hangs down the neck on to the upper anterior chest wall. When this occurs behind the sternum it is referred to as a *'retrosternal goitre or extension.'* If the lower pole of the gland is not palpable or if there is a history of difficulty in breathing, this possibility must be considered. Asking the patient to raise both arms and breathe in may cause a stridor – the *Pemberton's sign.*

Multinodular goitre

Multinodular goitre as the name indicates has multiple nodules. These are normally related to iodine deficiency. Solitary nodules undergo repeated cycles of hyperplasia and involution depending on the availability of iodine and finally manifest as multinodular goitre.

If there is a toxic thyroid nodule then medical or surgical management will be needed.

The indication for surgery is as outlined earlier and is determined by cosmesis and/or the presence or absence of compression. A *partial* or a *subtotal thyroidectomy* may be required.

In a benign solitary nodule, a *thyroid lobectomy* suffices. If the cytology suggests or confirms malignancy, a *total thyroidectomy* may be needed depending upon the size of the nodule.

Section 4: Hyperthyroidism

Hyperthyroidism – Grave's disease

When the gland becomes very active it produces an excess of thyroxine. TSH levels decrease. Excess thyroxine leads to an:

- Increase in BMR
- Weight loss
- Irritability
- Changes in the CVS
- Enhanced heat production leading to depletion of energy reserves such as liver glycogen and body fat
- Proptosis
- Exophthalmos and goitre

Graves's disease now tends to be managed medically rather than surgically; in assessing these patients' clinical signs affecting the ophthalmic and cardiac systems are important.

Robert Graves, in the mid-19th century, described a condition of exophthalmos associated with irregularities of the heart. We now know this to be an *autoimmune disorder,* triggered by environmental factors and is manifest more commonly in women.

Once confirmed the treatment tends to be medical with *carbimazole* and a β-*blocker* to decrease the sympathetic effects including tachycardia. In patients past their teens, it is reasonable to consider *radioiodine* when medical management fails; this cannot, however, be used in:

- The young
- Women in child-bearing age
- The pregnant

Surgery is reserved for those patients that fail to respond to medical management and in rare acute situations such as *'thyrocardiacs'* where the cardiac status needs urgent blockage of thyroid activity. These, by and large, tend to be 'historic' indications. When surgery is needed, a total thyroidectomy is usually required to prevent recurrence of Grave's disease; the risk of recurrence following *'subtotal thyroidectomy'* is around 5% and should be avoided. Surgical excision can also be considered in the presence of a toxic hot nodule causing thyrotoxicosis.

Section 5: Thyroid cancers

Thyroid cancers are rare. They are, however, one of the common endocrine malignancies. There are four types of thyroid cancer: three originate from the thyroid itself, and one arises from the parafollicular cells (C cells) that produce calcitonin. The embryologic origin of C cells is disputed but they share the properties of the neuroendocrine cells [similar to the adrenals and are, therefore, related to the amine precursor uptake and decarboxylation (APUD) group of cells].

The four cancers of the thyroid are:
1. Papillary thyroid carcinoma (PTC)
2. Follicular thyroid carcinoma (FTC)
3. Medullary thyroid carcinoma (MTC)
4. Anaplastic thyroid carcinoma (ATC)

Apart from these *lymphomas* and *secondaries* occur in the thyroid gland but these are not of thyroid origin.

Papillary thyroid carcinoma

This is the most common of thyroid cancers accounting for 80–85% of all thyroid cancers. It, like most thyroid disease, affects more women than men. This has the best prognosis among all thyroid cancers. It spreads predominantly via *lymphatics.*

Risk factors

- *Radiation exposure:* Increased numbers of cases were seen after Hiroshima and Nagasaki as well as Chernobyl. Treatment with radiotherapy for lymphoma during childhood may be a factor in a few.
- *Genetic factors* such as familial adenomatosis
- Presence of long-standing benign thyroid disease
- Excessive intake of iodine
- Obesity

Presentation

- They commonly present as a nodule in the thyroid gland with irregular edges.
- About 20–25% may present as a solitary cervical lymph node. It is used to be mistaken for *'lateral aberrant thyroid gland'* until it was realised that most were secondaries from a papillary carcinoma and not true aberrant thyroid tissue.
- Hoarseness of voice due to involvement of the recurrent laryngeal nerve may occur in a small proportion of patients.

Histologically, they have a *papillary pattern* with neoplastic changes surrounded by follicles.

Whenever a papillary pattern is seen even in the presence of follicles, it is normally treated as a papillary cancer.

Investigations

Ultrasound scan of the thyroid with fine-needle aspiration cytology (FNAC) assists in the diagnosis in most (**Table 1**). Cytology is reported as per the guidance of the *Royal College of Pathologists.*

Radio-isotope scanning if carried out will show these nodules to be cold nodules.

Thyroid function tests are likely to be normal.

Auto-antibody tests are carried out routinely and may also be normal.

CT and 18F-fluorodeoxyglucose (FDG)-positron emission tomography (PET)-CT are needed to establish the extent and spread of the disease in patients with tumours that are more advanced in size, T3 and T4 (**Table 2**).

Table 1 Role of thyroid ultrasound with fine-needle aspiration cytology (FNAC) in aiding diagnosis.	
THY category	**Description**
THY-1	Inadequate/Cystic lesion
THY-2	Benign and non-neoplastic
THY-3	Indeterminate and possible neoplasm
THY-4	Suspicious of malignancy
THY-5	Malignant

Table 2 TNM staging.	
Category	**Description**
T1	Tumour 2 cm or less
T2	Tumour 2–4 cm
T3	Tumour larger than 4 cm or grown just outside (T3b)
T4	Tumour involves adjacent structures
N0	No affected nodes
N1a	Nodes involved close to the gland
N1b	Nodes involved in both sides of the neck and chest
M0	No metastasis
M1	Presence of metastases

Treatment

The options include:

- Surgery with thyroxine replacement therapy
- Radio-iodine therapy with I-131
- Targeted therapy with tyrosine-kinase inhibitors

Surgery

- *Total thyroidectomy* and thyroxine suppressive therapy to push down TSH levels
- *Partial or hemi-thyroidectomy (T1 tumours)* where the affected lobe is resected along with the isthmus
- *Completion of thyroidectomy* where a previous partial thyroidectomy was carried out either for diagnosis or for treatment
- *Lymph node dissection* of the neck in case of lymph nodal involvement or prophylactic for high risk malignancies

Choice of operation needs discussion with the patient and MDT where it pertains. The type of thyroidectomy depends on:

- Underlying pathology (benign vs. malignant)
- Extent of disease (unilateral vs. bilateral)

- Risk of recurrence
- Patient factors (age, comorbidities)
- Surgeon experience

A ready rule of thumb is as follows:

Condition	Preferred surgery
Solitary thyroid nodule	Hemithyroidectomy
Papillary carcinoma ≤1 cm	Lobectomy
Papillary carcinoma >1 cm	Total thyroidectomy
Medullary carcinoma	Total thyroidectomy
Graves' disease	Total thyroidectomy
MNG (bilateral)	Total thyroidectomy
Recurrent disease	Total thyroidectomy
MNG, multinodular goitre	

The complications include:

- *Hoarseness* of voice due to inadvertent injury to recurrent laryngeal nerve; rarely bilateral injury leading to stridor. *Unilateral injury causes hoarseness and bilateral injury causes airway obstruction*
- *Parathyroid injury* normally ischaemic injury during total thyroidectomy and problems with hypocalcaemia
- External Laryngeal nerve supplies the cricothyroid muscle. It's injury leads to voice fatigue and loss of pitch that is important for singers. Avoidance of mass ligation of the superior thyroid artery and capsular dissection reduces the risk of injury.
- *Haemorrhage* and bleeding into a tight space in the neck causing difficulty in breathing. If it were to happen, the immediate action is to open the sutures in the neck in the ward and relieve the compression effect on the airways

Key points during thyroidectomy:

1. Identify the recurrent laryngeal nerve (RLN) in the tracheo-oesophageal groove and preserve it.
2. The RLN passes posterior to or between the branches of the inferior thyroid artery.
3. Dissection close to the thyroid capsule (capsular dissection) helps to preserve the vascularity of the parathyroids.
4. Avoid blind clamping, ligation, or cautery near the RLN.
5. Nerve stimulator is an adjunct, not a substitute, for nerve identification
6. Avoid haematoma with excellent haemostasis.

Radio active iodine therapy

As iodine is taken up by the thyroid tissue alone, treating hyperthyroid and differentiated thyroid cancers, such as papillary (**Table 3**) and follicular carcinoma (**Table 4**), with radioactive I-131 is effective. In case of thyroid cancers, it is useful for treating recurrence and residual disease as the radioactive iodine is taken up only by thyroid tissue. This results in destruction of the thyroid tissue.

Table 3 Papillary carcinoma.	
SEER stage	**5-year relative survival rate**
Localised	>99.5%
Regional	99%
Distant	74%
All stages combined	99.5%

Table 4 Follicular carcinoma.	
SEER stage	**5-year relative survival rate**
Localised	>99.5%
Regional	98%
Distant	67%
All stages combined	98%

External beam radiotherapy and chemotherapy may need consideration by the oncologists in select cases.

Replacement (suppressive) doses of thyroxine: This will be needed lifelong with monitoring of the TSH to ensure that the levels are kept very low.

SEER staging is a basic system from the National Cancer Institute Surveillance (NCIS, USA) and stands for surveillance, epidemiology and end results. It provides a system for assessing the burden of cancer and assists in understanding survival rates across different populations.

Follicular carcinoma

This is more common in women in their 30s. This is the second most common thyroid cancer accounting for 10–15% of all thyroid cancers. *The spread is haematogenous* unlike that of papillary cancer. It can metastasise to lungs and bones.

Treatment is very similar to that of papillary cancers. Total thyroidectomy and radioiodine therapy. External beam radiation may be necessary. Thyroxine replacement therapy will be needed life long and response with regular assessment of TSH levels.

Medullary carcinoma (Table 5)

- This is not truly thyroid cancer.
- Arises from the C cells and generally forms part of multiple endocrine neoplasia — MEN I and II.

Anaplastic carcinoma (Table 6)

Tends to affect the older age group. Survival is very poor with a very high mortality within a year of diagnosis. There is a limited role for surgery which includes the resection of isthmus of the thyroid gland if the patient has difficulty in breathing.

Table 5 Medullary thyroid cancer.

SEER stage	5-year relative survival rate
Localised	>99.5%
Regional	92%
Distant	43%
All stages combined	91%

Table 6 Anaplastic thyroid cancer.

SEER stage	5-year relative survival rate
Localised	39%
Regional	11%
Distant	4%
All stages combined	8%

Conclusion

Thyroid cancers are relatively uncommon. They are a diverse group with favourable outcomes when detected early. Advances in diagnostics, improved and targeted treatments have improved survival for most patients. Challenges of over treatment of indolent tumours and managing aggressive tumours remain a problem.

Chapter 9

Parathyroid disease and calcium metabolism

Srinivasan Ravi

Introduction

Three hormones regulate calcium levels and maintain calcium homeostasis.

- Parathormone (PTH)
- Calcitonin
- Calcitriol

Parathormone is secreted by the parathyroid glands that are located in the neck in intimate relationship to the thyroid gland. There are four parathyroid glands two of which are located behind each of the two lobes of the thyroid gland. In a small proportion of patients, they are aberrant, being located in the oesophagus, retro-sternum or elsewhere in the neck. They are quite tiny about the size of a pea. These tiny glands are responsible for maintaining the calcium/phosphorous homeostasis that is necessary to prevent fractures and maintain neuromuscular excitability.

Parathormone increases serum calcium levels: A feedback system releases PTH when the serum calcium level decreases. PTH, thus, works to increase calcium in serum. PTH moves calcium out of the bone by a *slow* and a *rapid process;* the slow process acts on *osteoclasts.* The rapid process pushes the calcium out of the *bone fluid* into the plasma.

PTH also acts on the *kidney* to retain calcium.

It increases absorption of calcium from the small bowel by stimulating the production of *calcitriol.*

Actions of parathormone

- Excitation – contraction coupling
- Excitation – secretion coupling
- Stability of excitable membranes
- Cardiac and smooth muscle activity
- Enzyme activity
- Coagulation
- Structure – bone, teeth, and connective tissue

Calcitonin is secreted by the *para-follicular C cells* in the thyroid gland.

Calcitonin decreases serum calcium levels

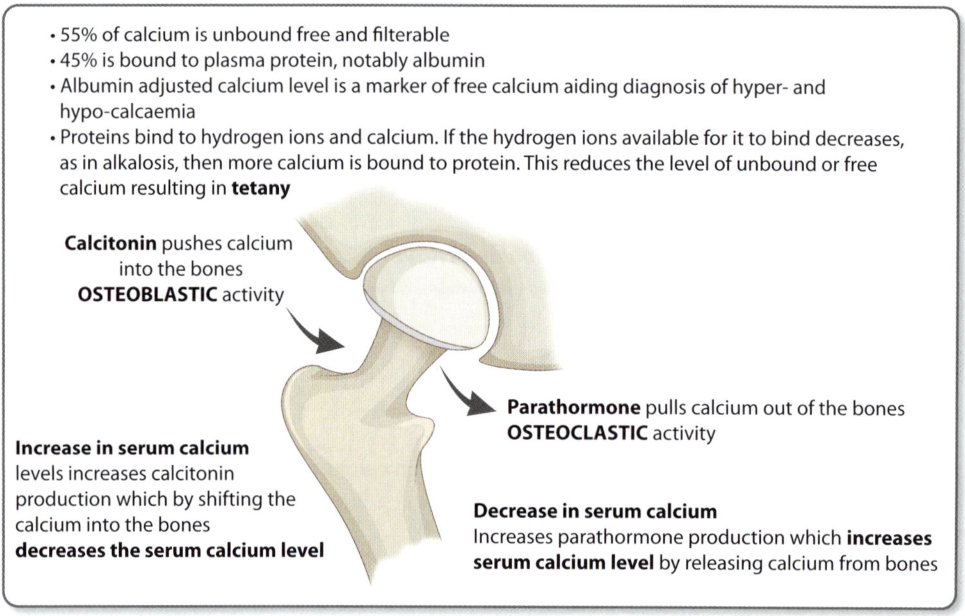

Figure 1 Calcium in plasma.

Calcitonin is released by a feedback system when the serum calcium increases (**Figure 1**). It works to decrease calcium levels in the serum. It stimulates osteoblasts and deposits calcium into the bone; it also inhibits osteoclasts thereby reducing calcium coming out of the bone.

Calcitriol is produced by the kidney. It is *the active form of vitamin D.*

Vitamin D is obtained from:

- Exposure to ultraviolet (UV) rays of the sun
- From foods
- From supplements

It is inactive. *Activation* requires two hydroxylations.

The first hydroxylation:

- Occurs in the liver
- The vitamin D is converted to 25-hydroxyvitamin D [25(OH)D]
- This is known as *'calcidiol.'*

The second hydroxylation:

- Occurs in the proximal convoluted tubule (PCT) of the kidneys
- Here, the physiologically active form, 1,25-dihydroxyvitamin D [1,25(OH)2D], is generated
- This is known as *'calcitriol'*

  Calcitriol elevates calcium levels by promoting absorption of calcium by enterocytes.

Calcitriol, thus, enhances the PTH effect on bone (**Table 1**).

Table 1 Parathormone – PTH versus calcitonin.

Parathormone – PTH	**Calcitonin**
Produced by parathyroid glands	Produced by parafollicular 'C' cells in the thyroid gland
Increases calcium levels	Decreases calcium levels
PTH production is increased in response to low-calcium levels	Calcitonin production is increased in response to high-calcium levels
Stimulates osteoclastic activity	*Inhibits* osteoclastic activity
Inhibits osteoblastic activity	*Stimulates* osteoblastic
PTH also acts on the kidney to retain calcium	
Stimulates calcitriol production and increases absorption of calcium from the small bowel	

Hyperparathyroidism

There are four parathyroid glands located behind the thyroid gland; occasionally they can be in other sites due to their embryological location during development.

Hyperthyroidism can be:

- Primary
- Secondary
- Tertiary

Primary hyperparathyroidism is due to:

- *Hyperplasia*: 10–15%
- *Adenoma:* 80–85%
- *Carcinoma*: 1%
- *Multiple endocrine neoplasia:*
  - *MEN-1:* Tumours occur in the *P*ituitary, *P*arathyroid, and *P*ancreas (PPP).
  - *MEN-2:* Tumours occur in the *P*arathyroid, *A*drenal, and *T*hyroid (PAT).

These are rare inherited autosomal dominant syndromes that need to be suspected when other endocrine organs are involved.

Secondary hyperparathyroidism is caused by chronic hypocalcaemia that stimulates compensatory parathyroid hormone (PTH) secretion. This is most commonly due to chronic renal disease. Other causes are malabsorption syndromes, chronic liver disease, dietary, vitamin D deficiency, and long term anti-convulsant therapy

Tertiary hyperparathyroidism is used to describe a chronically overactive parathyroid that has become autonomous. These present as hyperplasia rather than adenoma. They may follow renal transplantation for chronic renal failure.

Presenting features

Stones, bones, groans, and psychotic moans!

- Stones – renal stones
- Bones – osteoporosis and bone pain
- Groans – abdominal cramps
- Psychotic moans – neurological effects

Other symptoms

- Chronic fatigue syndrome
- Hypertension
- Atrial fibrillation

The *serum calcium level is elevated. The calcium level and symptoms do not have correlation.* It stands to reason, that if the PTH is elevated, it removes the calcium from the bone and moves it to circulation thus elevating the serum calcium levels.

Excess calcium can be deposited in atherosclerotic plaques causing hypertension.

The role of calcium in the 'excitation contraction process' can lead to conduction disorders in the heart and changes in the central nervous system (CNS) where calcium is a major player.

In the muscle, it causes fatigue and pain.

Denuding the bone of calcium causes bone problems including osteoporosis.

Excess elimination of calcium in the urine causes stones in the kidney.

If in any patient the serum calcium level is elevated, however slightly, it must be rechecked. If there is elevation in the presence of symptoms, PTH levels need to be checked.

Investigations

Localisation with:

- Ultrasound scan
- *Sestamibi scan* (MIBI scan) – a radio-isotope scan that uses sestamibi, a radioactive liquid that is taken up only by parathyroid tissue. The adenoma can then be localised by the uptake of the isotope which is viewed by a gamma camera.

A dual-energy X-ray absorptiometry (DEXA) scan can be done to define the level of osteoporosis.

Surgical treatment

The patients are best treated in a centre with experience. Minimally invasive focussed surgery with a small incision in the neck is appropriate for an adenoma once it is isolated by imaging. Generally, an adenoma presents as a solitary adenoma that causes the problem, but it can also be due to multiple or ectopic adenomas. When there are multiple adenomas or hyperplasia, then a total parathyroidectomy with removal of all the parathyroid glands may be needed despite the possible complications that follow with the calcium metabolism.

Postoperatively, bone pain improves immediately. These patients need to be monitored for calcium levels as, occasionally, the bones being denuded of calcium for some time deplete the serum calcium by taking up all available calcium leading to the *hungry bone syndrome*. These patients will need intravenous calcium and specialist care.

Few patients may need vitamin D and calcium if rendered hypo-parathyroid.
Re-operation may be needed in the few (5% cases) with persistent or recurrent HPT that usually results from double adenomas or multiglandular hyperplasia.

Secondary hyperparathyroidism is due to poor renal function with retained phosphate bonding with calcium. This may only just lower the calcium but over time this stimulates the production of PTH leading to secondary hyper-parathyroid disorder. Secondary HPT is usually managed medically. Surgery is required in only 3–5% of patients.

Conclusion

Parathyroid glands maintain calcium-phosphorus balance via PTH. Hyperparathyroidism causes hypercalcaemia and bone disease. Hypoparathyroidism, mostly due to iatrogenic injury causes hypocalcaemia with neuromuscular irritability. Calcium homeostasis is central not only to bone health but also to maintenance of neuromuscular instability and activity of the cardiac and central nervous systems.

Chapter 10

Nutrition of the surgical patient

Srinivasan Ravi

Introduction

Nutritional requirements of the surgical patient are variable and are affected by the complex processes controlling the metabolic response to surgical trauma, the magnitude and duration of that trauma and the characteristics of the individual that sustained that trauma, such the basal metabolic rate (BMR).

Section 1: Assessment and need of nutritional support

Nutritional assessment must be considered for all patients, not only those defined as being malnourished by any of the following criteria using the '*Malnutrition Universal Screening Tool (MUST)*' that was developed and launched by BAYPEN in 2003. MUST scoring is done routinely in the NHS. National Institute of Health and Care Excellence (NICE) recommends screening at the following times:

- On admission to the hospital and weekly thereafter
- On admission to care homes
- At initial outpatient appointments
- At initial registration with general practice surgery

The MUST score has five steps.

- *Step 1*: BMI score
  - Score 0: BMI > 20
  - Score 1: BMI 18.5–20
  - Score 2: BMI < 18.5
- *Step 2*: Unintentional weight loss score
  - Score 0: < 5% weight loss in the last 3–6 months
  - Score 1: 5–10% weight loss in the last 3–6 months
  - Score 2: > 10% weight loss in the last 3–6 months
- *Step 3*: Acute disease effect score
  - Score 0: Patient without serious illness but has had little or no nutritional intake for 5 or more days
  - Score 2: Patient with serious illness but has had little or no nutritional intake for 5 or more days
- *Step 4*: Total the score

- *Step 5*: Determine the risk category
  - Medium risk - score of 1
  - High risk score of 2 or more

The malnourished patient has:
- Body mass index (BMI) of <18.5 kg/m^2
- Unintentional weight loss > 10% within the last 3–6 months
- Body mass index of <20 kg/m^2 and unintentional weight loss > 5% within the last 3–6 months.

To this can be added:
- Patients who have eaten little or nothing for >5 days
- Patients who are likely to eat little or nothing for 5 days or longer
- Patients with a poor absorptive capacity
- Patients with high nutrient losses
- Patients with increased nutritional needs from causes such as catabolism

Body mass index or BMI

The MUST score includes assessment of BMI. Simply put, BMI is an index that tells us the ratio of the weight a person carries for the height. An adult's weight in kilograms divided by their height in metres squared gives the BMI for that individual. For example, A BMI of 25 means 25 kg/m^2.

BMI ranges

For most adults, an ideal BMI is in the 18.5–24.9 kg/m^2 range.

For children and young people aged 2–18, the BMI calculation takes into account age and gender as well as height and weight.

If the BMI is:
- Below 18.5 - underweight range
- Between 18.5 and 24.9 kg/m^2 - 'healthy' weight range
- Between 25 and 29.9 kg/m^2 - overweight range
- 30 kg/m^2 or over - obese range

BMR or the basal metabolic rate

This is the number of calories needed to perform the basic activities such as maintaining circulation, breathing, cell production and destruction, etc.

It is affected by the lean muscle mass of the individual as muscle burns more calories than fat. The BMR of an individual is dependent on:
- Body composition
- Age
- Gender
- Genetic make up

BMR is the prime component of the energy that is expended by the body.

Calories burnt/day or *energy expenditure* is a sum of:
- BMR (60–70%) – ion activity, protein building, recycling metabolites, etc.
- Activity thermogenesis (15–30%) – resting and exercise
- Thermic effect of digestion (10%)

Factors that increase energy expenditure in surgical patients:
- Elective surgery – 10%
- Trauma – 10–30%
- Sepsis/Infections – 50–80%
- Burns – 100%

The progressive increase in energy requirements is met by utilising or burning carbohydrate, fat and proteins. Once the carbohydrate and fat are used up then the body turns to proteins to meet the increased expenditure.

Points of note in the nutrition of the surgical patient

- Malnutrition is common in surgical patients
- Obese patients can be malnourished
- Poor nutrition prolongs stay due to problems with postoperative infection and poor wound healing
- Low BMI is a contributor to poor recovery
- Very high BMI makes surgery difficult and increases intraoperative complications
- Serum albumin may not be a marker of poor nutrition. It is an important acute phase reactant
- Obesity disadvantages the surgeon and the patient

Successful outcomes following surgery may depend upon good nutritional status. The nutritional status of patients undergoing any type of surgery must be assessed. Elective surgery permits an opportunity to ensure that the patient is nutritionally fit. Sometimes as in patients with gastric or pancreatic malignancy or Crohn's disease this might well-nigh be impossible without preoperative prehabilitation with nutritional support.

Section 2: Physiology

Starvation and impact on metabolism

Surgical management of patients includes a period of starvation for patients and hence recollection of the basic physiology of starvation will assist in the understanding of the impact of starvation on patients.

The brain and the red cells can only use glucose as their source of energy.

As hunter gatherers, homo sapiens were exposed to prolonged periods of starvation. Storage of glucose for use during times of lack of availability of food, therefore, led to the evolutionary adaptation to deal with such situations. The adaptation over time included two important mechanisms of:

1. Gylcogenolysis
2. Gluconeogenesis

Glycogenolysis

The body stores glucose as glycogen in the liver. The glycogen is released by the liver as glucose during short periods of starvation by the process of glycogenolysis, which converts stored glycogen to glucose, to maintain the blood sugar levels.

Glycogen stores are depleted within 24 hours.

Gluconeogenesis

If the starvation is prolonged the body resorts to gluconeogenesis, the *synthesis of 'new' glucose from amino acids* such as alanine and glycine to maintain the blood sugar levels. In situations of stress and starvation, glucocorticoids as the 'gluco' implies facilitates gluconeogenesis. This hormone also assists *glucogon* in the process of gluconeogenesis.

The brain can use only glucose as it is water soluble and thus able to cross the 'blood-brain' barrier where it takes part in the energy transfer citric acid cycle (Krebs cycle) and generates adenosine triphosphate (ATP).

Once the glucose storage is depleted, gluconeogenesis can assist in providing glucose but there is also an evolutionary need to protect the protein in the body as they are necessary for enzyme reactions and muscle function.

Saving protein – the golden rule

This is done by switching the substrate to ketones from glucose as the source of energy for the metabolism of the brain.

Switching to breaking down fats initially produces fatty acids and acetyl-CoA that can enter the Krebs cycle.

After 3 days of starvation an excess of acetyl-CoA builds up with slowing of the Krebs cycle. This enters the liver where it is converted to ketones.

There are three ketone bodies:

1. Acetoacetate
2. 3-β-hydroxybutyrate
3. Acetone the least abundant

The brain can use ketones as they are able to pass through the blood-brain barrier. This process protects the utilisation of protein as the brain switches from utilisation of glucose to utilising ketones as a source of energy. This preserves the much-needed proteins.

Primacy of the integrity of the intestinal mucosa

The mucosa of the intestine thrives on nutrients obtained from contact with the ingest. It serves as a barrier to pathogens from the diet while at the same time allowing for absorption of nutrients and fluid (**Table 1**).

Table 1 Absorption of nutrients in the small and large bowel.

Duodenum	**Iron and calcium**
Jejunum	Sugars, amino acids and fatty acids
Ileum	B12 and bile salts
Colon	Water and electrolytes

The cells lining the intestines include:

- The enterocytes
- Paneth cells
- The goblet cells
- T cells
- B cells
- The dendritic cells
- Macrophages
- Innate lymphoid cells

Lack of mucosal contact with nutrients leads to lymphoid tissue atrophy, immune-system functional decline, and intensification in bacterial translocation. Currently, it is assumed that *microbiome* is one of the body organs that has a significant impact on health. The composition of microbiome is not affected by age, sex, or place of residence, although it changes rapidly after diet modification. The composition of the microbiome is determined by enterotype, which is specific for each organism. It has a significant impact on the risk of diabetes, cancer, atherosclerosis, and other diseases.

The intestinal immune system – This is an exquisite system. Toll-like receptors are located on the apical surface of the intestinal epithelium. They collect pathogen-associated molecular patterns and transfer them to antigen-presenting cells. Based on obtained information, gut–associated lymphoid tissue (GALT) differentiates commensal bacteria from pathogenic and either tolerates or destroys them. GALT is composed of lymphoid aggregates, Peyer's patches, isolated lymphoid follicles diffusely distributed along the lamina propria, and intraepithelial lymphocytes. It is estimated that GALT contains approximately 70% of total immune system cells.

These cells are involved not only in the absorption of nutrients but also in innate immunity. The mucosal barrier secreted by goblet cells assists in reduction of inflammatory response to pathogens in food while the dendritic cell assists in pattern recognition of pathogenic antigens. The amazing arrangement of this array of cells in the mucosa houses a large part of the immune system in the GALT and provides a neural enteral network ENS. The enteric nervous system is the "little brain" of the gut. It consists of two main plexuses: The myenteric plexus (Auerbach's plexus, located between muscle layers) and the submucosal plexus (Meissner's plexus, located just beneath the mucosal layer). This extensive network of over 100 million nerve cells lines the GIT from the esophagus to the rectum.

This intricate neuro-immune network allows the body to coordinate a complex response to maintain gut barrier integrity and defend against pathogens, involving both immune defense mechanisms and changes in gut function (e.g. increased motility to expel harmful substances). This system can be breached by infections, inflammation, medication, and surgery leading to bacterial transgression through the mucosal barrier.

Reasons for fluid accumulation in ileus

- *Secreted fluids from:*
  - Oral cavity – saliva

  - Gastric secretions
  - Intestinal secretions – succus entericus
- *Absence of peristaltic force that is controlled by a combination of:*
  - Enteric nervous system – Auerbach's plexus, etc.
  - Autonomic nervous system – sympathetic and parasympathetic

Section 3: Types of nutritional support

- Enteral nutrition
- Parenteral nutrition

Enteral nutrition

If the gastrointestinal tract is available for use, then use it!

It is the most preferred way of providing nutrition. Enteral nutrition (EN) also serves to preserve the integrity of the intestinal mucosa which derives its nutrition from diet. When this is denied, the villi atrophy and lose their activity. The presence of the villi increases the surface area of the intestines available for absorption. In the absence of enterally derived nutrition, the atrophy of the villi leads to a reduction in surface area available for absorption. This is one of the reasons why some patients get diarrhoea on re-introduction of enteral feeding after a period of suspension. Preservation of the mucosa retains the activity in the villi. Furthermore, enteral feeding has less complications than parenteral nutrition.

Traditionally, patients were treated with 'nil by mouth' during the early post laparotomy period. The result of early enteral feeding is equivocal with some studies suggesting benefits with respect to wound healing and length of stay while others show no benefit. Provision of early enteral nutrition may provide more energy that promotes healing. According to a recent Cochrane review update, which reviewed 17 RCTs with the total number of 1,437 participants the authors concluded that 'early enteral feeding may lead to a reduced postoperative length of stay; however, cautious interpretation must be taken due to substantial heterogeneity and low-quality evidence. For all other outcomes postoperative complications, mortality, adverse events, and quality of life (QoL) the findings are inconclusive'.

In the early postoperative period, however, re-introduction of oral feeding must be done with caution as vomiting may occur. Numbers needed to harm (NNH) is 19 as per the recent Cochrane review.

Methods of using the enteral system:

- Oral supplementation
- Nasogastric feeding
- Fine bore feeding
- *Gastrostomy:*
  - Surgical – open procedure
  - Percutaneous endoscopic-guided (PEG)
  - PEGJ – when the PEG is placed in the jejunum
- Jejunostomy for distal intestinal feeding

Delivery of enteral nutrition

Ideally suited for situations where long-term enteral feeding is needed as in patients with oesophageal pathology or with low fistula of the small bowel. A discussion with a clinician with a special interest is needed. In some hospitals, there will be nutritional leads and dietitians who will assist in the planning and delivery of enteral nutrition.
The planning and prescription of enteral nutrition takes into consideration:

- Type of tube to be used for feeding
- Location of the tip of the tube
- Different modes of access
- The total quantity of fluid per day
- Total calories needed per day. Critically ill patients need more calories
- Macro- and micronutrients needed
- Proteins/carbohydrate needed per kilogram of body weight
- Frequency of feeding
- Timing of feeding – i.e. overnight and intermittent
- Types of fluid to be used:
  - *Standard* – non-hydrolysed macronutrients for patients with a normal gastrointestinal (GI) tract
  - *Elemental* or peptide – hydrolysed macronutrients for those with malabsorption
  - *Carbohydrate controlled* for diabetics with a higher fibre and fat but less carbohydrate

Complications of enteral feeding

- *Aspiration of gastric contents:* This can be *silent* as in intubated patients in the ITU or *overt* when clinically obvious.
  - Occurs with nasogastric as well as gastrostomy feeding
  - More common in elderly
  - Poor oral hygiene and decreased salivary flow can be contributing factors
  - Large bore nasogastric tube (NGT) may permit aspiration through an open gastro-oesophageal junction
  - Low residual volume (RV) in stomach during enteral feeding (<100 mL every 4 hours) may contribute to a reduction in risk of aspiration. Some studies have shown that aspiration may occur irrespective of the RV.
  - Reduction in risk can be achieved by *vertical nursing* while feeding or retaining an inclination of 45° for an hour after feeding
  - *Aspiration can lead to:*
    - *Chemical pneumonitis* when the stomach contents are acidic
    - Interstitial or *aspiration pneumonia* with bacterial infection
    - *Atelectasis* due to solid particles in aspirate

Checking gastric residual volume (RV) every 4 hours and maintaining a residual level of <100 mL are usually advocated during tube feeding. However, it has been shown that the frequencies of regurgitation and aspiration are similar over a wide range of RV from 0 to 400 mL. Hence, RV is not a reliable marker of aspiration. On the other hand, large-bore nasogastric (NG) tubes may increase the risk of aspiration of gastric contents by interfering with normal lower oesophageal sphincter.

- *Refeeding syndrome:* This is a potentially fatal fluid and electrolyte shifts that can occur on initiating feeding in malnourished patients. This can occur in patients–
  - Not fed for 5 days
  - Manifests within 5 days of onset of enteral feeding
  - Patients have low phosphate, magnesium and potassium
  - May have fluid shifts leading to fatigue, confusion and cardiac failure
  - High index of suspicion is needed to detect this
  - It can be avoided by restriction of calories in the feed initially to 1,000 calories on the first day – *start low and go slow*
- *Malposition of tube:* When a fine bore tube is used, its position must be verified by radiology prior to initiating feeding lest the tube lodges in the bronchial tree.
- *Complications of surgical gastrostomy:*
  - Wound-related complications such as dehiscence and infection
  - Haemorrhage
  - Slippage of gastrostomy tube
  - Peritonitis due to leak around the tube or misplacement
  - Complications arising from anaesthesia
- *Complications of percutaneous endoscopic gastrosotomy (PEG) tubes:*
  - As for gastrostomy
  - Tube malfunction
  - Leakage of feed around the tube

Nutritional requirement

- *Water:* Most 'feeds' are water-based. This needs to be calculated for every patient. As a ready rule of thumb 2,500–3,500 mL/day is recommended
- *Macronutrient:*
  - *Carbohydrate* energy provided is 4 kcal/g. Approximately – 300 g/day
  - *Protein* energy provided is 4 kcal/g. Approximately – 90 g/day
  - *Fat* energy provided is 9 kcal/g. Approximately – 55 g/day
- *Calorie requirement per day:*
  - Males 2,500 kcal/day
  - Females 2,000 kcal/day

- *Micronutrients:*
  - Vitamins
  - Minerals
  - Trace elements

Parenteral nutrition

Parenteral nutrition is defined as nutrition that is provided by a route other than enteral that is on a *par with enteral feeding.* This is *needed when the enteral route is not available* for provision of nutrition.

- Peripheral line feeding
- Central line feeding
- Immune enhancing nutrition

The nutrition is provided through veins. As the fluid that is given is hyperosmotic the peripheral veins develop thrombophlebitis within days and, hence, traditionally central veins are used.

In some situations, where short-term parenteral feeding of <2 weeks is anticipated, peripheral veins may be used for access. This is referred to as peripheral venous parenteral nutrition – *PPN* as opposed to *TPN* or total parenteral nutritionthrough the central veins.

The National Institute of Care excellence in the UK, NICE recommends starting parenteral feeding at no >50% of estimated needs for the first 24–48 hours with close monitoring of progress.

Parenteral nutrition can be used till the nutritional status becomes stable and enteral feeding can be re-established.

Access for parenteral nutrition

Central venous catheter: These cannulate the large veins such as the internal jugular, subclavian and femoral veins preferably under ultrasound guidance where this facility is available. The central venous catheter is advanced and placed in the superior or inferior vena cava and the position confirmed radiologically.

In patients needing long-term enteral feeding, >30 days, tunnelled subclavian lines are preferred.

PICC lines: These are peripherally introduced central catheters. They use the basilic or the brachial veins for access and are advanced to the superior vena cava.

All lines placed in the central veins and used for feeding must:

- Be placed under *aseptic* conditions, preferably in surgical theatres
- Be placed by healthcare teams skilled in the placement of these lines
- Have the position of the central line confirmed radiologically prior to initiating feeding
- Be always handled under *sterile conditions* – i.e. with surgical gloves and cleansing before and after every use
- Be dedicated to the sole use of nutritional feeding. A free lumen of a multi-lumen catheter can be used if it is dedicated to feeding

Section 4: Complications of central lines

These can be classified as follows:

- *Insertion-related:*
  - Haemorrhage/Haematoma
  - Arrhythmia
  - Pneumothorax
  - Injury to major arterial vessels
  - Air embolism
  - Wrong location of tip

These are procedure-related and avoidable with utmost care and ultrasonic imaging; however, multiple attempts at placements can lead to increased risk of complications.

- *Catheter-related:*
  - Site-related infection
  - Line infection – 'pus somewhere, pus nowhere, pus in the lines' is the new adage!
  - Catheter thrombosis
  - Venous thrombosis and embolism
  - Loss of catheter sites in patients requiring life or long-term usage
  - Sepsis
- *Feed-related:*
  - *Metabolic complications:*
    - Electrolyte imbalance
    - Hyper-/hypoglycaemia
    - Dehydration
    - Micronutrient deficiencies
  - *Hepatic complications:*
    - Elevated bilirubin/alkaline phosphatase due to cholestasis
    - Fibrosis/cirrhosis in patients using TPN for long term
  - *Candida infections* can arise from TPN use.

Attention to the nutritional status of the surgical patients may assist in the progress of the patient in the perioperative phase. Prolonged preoperative starvation is detrimental as much as early oral feeding is beneficial when used with due attention and care.

Enteral route of feeding where possible is the preferred route of feeding.

Addressing patients at nutritional risk at the outset and addressing it early will enhance recovery.

Chapter 11

Metabolic response to trauma

Srinivasan Ravi

Section 1: Introduction

Trauma in any form sets off an amazing cascade of response that is geared to meet the increased oxygen and energy demands imposed on the system. This demand is proportional to the trauma sustained.

The response is evolutionary. It is orchestrated by the pituitary and is primarily an endocrine response. There is also an immunological component to it as the body gears itself to ward off intruders.

The response induces tachycardia and tachypnoea. This helps to meet the increased demand for oxygen that is generated by the stress induced by any type of trauma. The endocrine response, increases the production of both catecholamines and cortisol (The 2 C's). Increasing respiratory rate makes available more oxygen for distribution to the tissues.

Increasing the heart rate enables the pump to supply oxygen to the tissues.

Cuthbertson in 1932 studied four patients and defined the phases of this response that has been subsequently referred to as the Ebb and Flow phases.

Egdhal, in 1950s, showed this response to be a *neurologically mediated sympathetic response.* He injured the legs of dogs while retaining the sciatic nerve. Samples were collected from adrenal veins and these showed elevated adrenaline and glucocorticoids. When the sciatic nerve was divided there was no change in the levels of adrenaline and glucocorticoids.

Section 2: Physiology

Endocrine response has three components:

1. Activation of the sympathetic system
2. The pituitary response
3. The insulin resistance

There are three phases:

1. Ebb phase
2. Flow phase
3. Anabolic phase

The term *'ebb phase'* denotes the period when the body retracts into a shell in an attempt to hold on to what its environment.

The *'flow phase'* refers to its attempt to overflow with supply of much-needed energy by mobilising resources to meet the requirements. This is akin to any natural calamity when the government initially assesses the damage (ebb) and then meets the needs (flow) with increased supply of food and water, etc.

The rebuilding – *the anabolic phase* occurs later.

- *Ebb phase* – that sets in immediately after surgery or trauma and *lasts for up to 2 days* during which time the body assesses the damage. It attempts to protect the existing resources by homeostasis, maintaining perfusion decreasing energy expenditure and retaining urinary nitrogen.
- Flow phase – *lasts from 2 to 7 days.* It is a survival response that can be defined as an 'all or none' reaction. This catabolic response attempts to mobilise the flow of substrate to meet the needs.
- Anabolic phase – this follows the flow phase. Rebuilding process *begins by 3–8 days after elective surgery,* but it is delayed after sepsis or major trauma or burns.

*The key aspects of the metabolic response to injury (**Figure 1**):*

- Immediate protective response
- Net effect is the increase of catabolic hormones
- Normally, there is a controlled catabolic response
- Catabolyses carbohydrate/protein/fats
- It is an evolutionary response as the injured animal uses body fuel, salt and water. It survives or dies without food
- Lastly, an anabolic response that rebuilds

The catabolic response is mediated primarily by adrenaline.

The catabolic response encashes the body's 'silver' made up of adipose tissue and muscle mass. Burning these makes available the 'energy' for the immediate needs. It is driven by catecholamines, glucagon, corticosteroids, and insulin resistance although it is predominantly an adrenal generated response. This process it has been said 'sells the silver to raise funds to

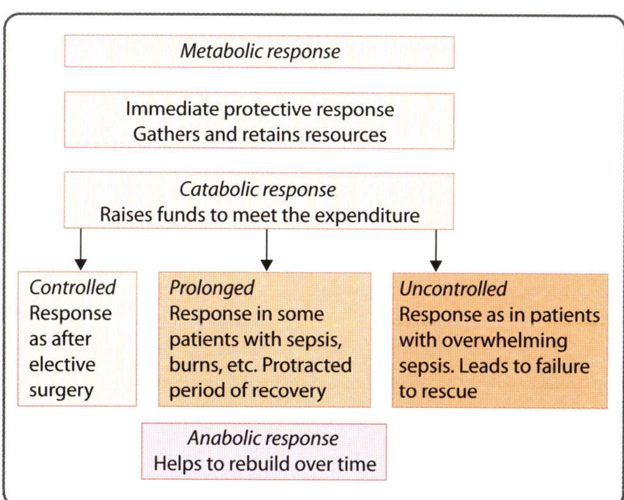

Figure 1 Metabolic response to injury.

meet the immediate expenditure' needed to manage the crisis. When uncontrolled, much like a gambler, the sale of silver goes to extremes to the detriment of the individual.

The resistance to insulin, an anabolic hormone, opposes the anabolic response.

The anabolic response is mostly mediated by the prime anabolic hormone, insulin as well as growth hormone, thyroxine and testosterone.

The anabolic response increases uptake by the injured tissue of:

- Glucose
- Amino acids
- Fats

This rebuilding response starts in 3–8 days depending on the magnitude of the trauma.

It is delayed after:

- Sepsis
- Burns
- Major trauma

The immunological response is based on:

- Cytokine production – from activated leucocytes
- Acute phase reactants
- Neutrophil leucocytosis

Section 3: Acute phase proteins response

The acute phase response (APR) is a prominent systemic reaction of the organism to local or systemic disturbances in its homeostasis caused by infection, tissue injury, trauma or surgery, neoplastic growth or immunological disorders (*Gordon and Koy).*

The acute phase proteins (APP) can be positive or negative. Within a few hours after infection or injury, the pattern of protein synthesis by the liver is drastically altered resulting in an increase of some blood proteins, the *positive APPs*. Hepatic messenger ribonucleic acid (mRNA) upregulation of those APPs is associated with a decrease in synthesis of normal blood proteins, like transferrin and *albumin,* which represent the *negative APPs.*

This is the reason that the albumin levels drop after major operations and sepsis.

The changes initiated by the acute phase response are:

- Increased cytokine production (by leucocytes)
- Increased interleukin 6 (IL-6) production
- Increased production of liver acute phase proteins such as immunoglobulins
- Increase in C-reactive protein (CRP). CRP is not just a marker of inflammation; it contributes to host defense by opsonisation and complement activation
- Increase in fibrinogen
- Decrease in albumin levels – a negative acute phase protein

> The acute phase response (APR) is a prominent systemic reaction of the organism to local or systemic disturbances in its homeostasis caused by infection, tissue injury, trauma or surgery, neoplastic growth or immunological disorders.

Continued...

Continued...

Pro-inflammatory cytokines are released at the site of insult, and the vascular system and inflammatory cells are activated. These, in turn, are associated with production of more cytokines and other inflammatory mediators which diffuse to the extracellular fluid compartment and circulate in the blood.

The cytokines activate receptors on different target cells leading to a systemic reaction resulting in activation of the hypothalamic–pituitary–adrenal axis, and reduction of growth hormone secretion.

Changes can be measured in the laboratory such as:

- A decrease in leucocyte numbers in blood
- Increased values of adrenocorticotrophic hormone (ACTH) and glucocorticoids
- Activation of the complement system and blood coagulation system
- Decreased serum levels of calcium, zinc and iron
- A change in concentration of several plasma proteins, the acute phase proteins (APPs) largely due to a changed hepatic metabolism.

Section 4: The hypothalamo-hypophysial axis (Figure 2)

The endocrine response is generated by the pathways shown in **Figure 3**.

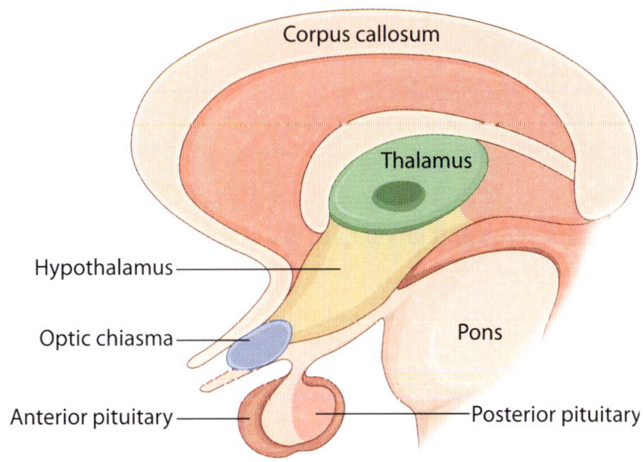

Hypothalamo-hypophyseal **portal system** is a system of micro circulation at the base of the brain that links the hypothalamus and the anterior pituitary. The posterior pituitary is linked directly by neurons. Note the proximity of the pituitary to the optic chiasma

HPA: Hypothalamo–pituitary–adrenal axis
regulates adrenal corticosteroid response
HPT: Hypothalamo–pituitary–thyroxine axis
regulates thyroxine levels
HPG: Hypothalamo–pituitary–gonadal axis
regulates sex hormone levels

Figure 2 Control of the endocrine orchestra.

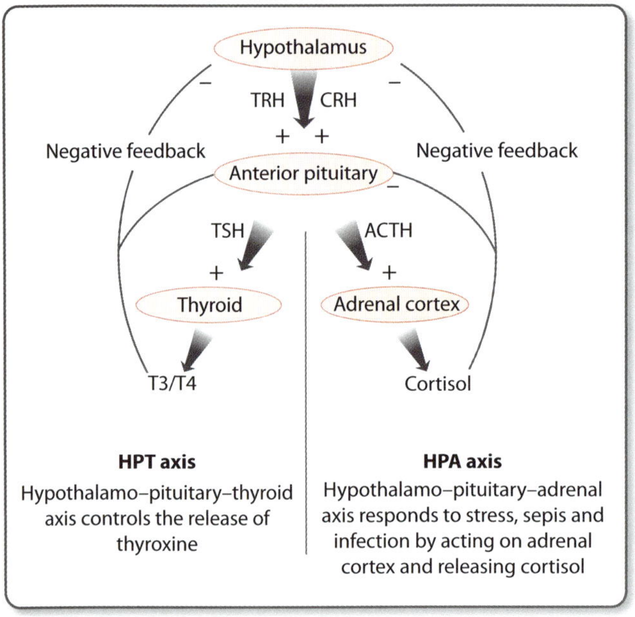

Figure 3 Endocrine response pathway.

ACTH, adrenocorticotropic hormone; CRH, corticotropin-releasing hormone; TRH, thyrotropin-releasing hormone; TSH, thyroid-stimulating hormone.

Section 5: Insulin resistance

Insulin resistance is defined as a condition in which the body fails to respond appropriately to the action of insulin, thus pushing up the blood sugar levels. It leads to decreased absorption of sugar by muscles, fat and liver cells. This leads to increased blood sugar levels which in turn stimulates the production of more insulin by the pancreas in a bid to promote absorption. Thus, the blood sugar rises, and the insulin level rises, and the body is unable to use the excess sugar leading to a situation akin to starvation. Therefore, there is 'poverty in the midst of plenty.'

- Insulin is an anabolic hormone
- Assists in utilisation of carbohydrate, proteins and fat that are the building blocks of healing
- Insulin resistance sets in rapidly after all and any type of surgery
- It lasts for a variable length of time depending on the magnitude of the operation
- It is a *fundamental response to stress*

When there are complications after elective surgery or in the presence of a major insult to the system such as sepsis, the resistance to insulin is:

- Greater
- Longer
- Prolongs the catabolic phase
- Prevents anabolism setting in

Olle Ljungvist, a key proponent of the enhanced recovery (ERAS) or fast track surgery, makes the following points about insulin resistance:

- Insulin resistance is proportional to the magnitude of the operation
- In major laparotomies, up to 90% of insulin sensitivity may be lost after surgery

- Even after moderate surgery this change can last for a week
- *Clear relationship exists between insulin resistance and postoperative complications, particularly infections*
- By prolonging recovery, insulin resistance may be harmful
- Hyperglycaemia after surgery is a direct result of insulin resistance
- Complications can be avoided if hyperglycaemia is controlled
- Regardless of perioperative diabetic state, less insulin resistance resulted in fewer complications
- *Keeping insulin resistance under control seems to be beneficial*
- Reduction or prevention of insulin resistance can be achieved as in ERAS by:
  - Preoperative carbohydrate loading instead of fasting moving the patient to the 'fed' or anabolic state
  - Using epidural anaesthesia before the onset of surgery
  - Continuing pain relief postoperatively
  - Early enteral feeding to avoid starvation-induced insulin resistance
- *Reduction in insulin resistance reduces time to recovery*

For critically ill patients after major trauma or sepsis, most evidence supports maintaining blood glucose in the range of 140–180 mg/dL (7.8–10 mmol/L). Tighter control (110–144 mg/dL or 6.1–8 mmol/L) may reduce infection risk but increases hypoglycaemia. Current best practice is to avoid uncontrolled hyperglycaemia (>180 mg/dL) while minimising hypoglycaemia, aiming for a moderate target of 100–150 mg/dL with an upper limit of 180 mg/dL depending on patient risk and institutional protocols. In practical terms this means:

- *Avoid extremes*: <70 mg/dL (hypoglycaemia) and >180 mg/dL (hyperglycaemia)
- *Preferred range*: 140–180 mg/dL for most critically ill patients
- *Individualisation*: Some trauma/sepsis protocols use 100–150 mg/dL if close monitoring is feasible

Conclusion

The metabolic response to trauma, generated by the integrated actions of the hormonal and immune systems, is crucial for survival as it reallocates energy substrates, maintains glucose availability to vital organs, enhances immune defense through acute-phase responses, and supports wound healing and tissue repair while restoring homeostasis.

Chapter 12

General plastic surgery

Srinivasan Ravi

Introduction

The skin is the largest organ of the body. It has a superficial layer, the epidermis, and a deeper layer the dermis that has the blood vessels, nerves and fibroblasts. A deeper layer, subcutis has the collagen and fat cells. Deep to this is the subcutaneous tissue.

The epidermis has three layers:

1. Stratum corneum containing the protein keratin and dead layers that flake off. Keratin provides 'the water proofing'.
2. Keratinocytes layer of living cells that mature and move superficially
3. Basal layer where new cells are laid out

Skin and subcutaneous lumps

Superficially, palpable lumps can be classified as being:

- Intradermal
- Subcutaneous
- Subfascial
- Intramuscular

Lumps can arise from structures in the different planes.

- The dermis – *pilar or 'sebaceous' cysts,* implantation dermoid or congenital angular dermoid
- Subcutaneous fat – *lipoma*
- Nerves – *neurofibroma*
- Lymphoidal tissue – lymph nodes

Dermal lumps

These are in the dermis of the skin and not in the subcutaneous tissue. They are, therefore, not mobile. Pilar or sebaceous cysts may have a punctum; the edge is well-defined. These commonly occur in parts of the body with hair and when these cysts become large the hair over the cyst is typically absent. They arise from the pilar glands at the root of the hair follicle but are commonly called sebaceous cysts rather than correctly, pilar cysts.

Management

Surgery is required if the cyst is painful or increasing in size. On occasions, the cyst can get infected, and the contents may discharge spontaneously leaving nothing more than a residual nubbin of tissue. This can be left alone or excised if necessary. Normally, these lumps are excised under local anaesthetic infiltration. An elliptical incision is made around the punctum and skin flaps developed over the cyst. If a small quantity of local anaesthesia is infiltrated in the plane between the cyst and the skin without puncturing the cyst it facilitates dissection. A plane is also developed deep to the cyst and the cyst can then be shelled out like a pea in a pod. Very small cysts that are adherent to the skin can be excised in toto along with the skin if the defect can be approximated easily. The skin can be approximated with subcuticular suture, or skin glue, if there is no tension and with interrupted sutures if there is tension. As these cysts are most often present in the scalp there may be a tendency to increased vascularity leading to bleeding. The need for meticulous haemostasis is, therefore, paramount.

Lipoma

These are commonly subcutaneous. They have a well-defined edge that slips under the palpating hand unlike the dermal cysts. Classically, when they are in the subcutaneous plane the mobility is present in all directions, unlike a neurofibroma that moves only along the plane of the nerve; however, lipoma may occur in different planes under the skin. Lipoma in the back tends to be large and tends to extend to deeper planes. When they extend deep they are not very mobile as there are multiple septae that radiate from the skin to the deep fascia making the dissection difficult. In the back, if located in the midline they may also extend into the spinal canal.

Locations of lipoma:

- Subcutaneous
- Subfascial
- Intermuscular
- Submuscular
- Intra-articular

Management

Mere presence of a lipoma is not an indication for surgery. The duration of the lipoma and its behaviour determine the indication for surgery.

Many lipomata tend to grow slowly and remain asymptomatic over years. If there is, however, a change in its rate of growth or there is an increase in symptoms such as pain, then surgical intervention may be necessary. The larger lipoma especially the ones in the back may require a short general anaesthesia for their removal.

Neurofibroma (Table 1)

These are benign neural sheath tumours. As they arise from the nerves, their mobility is restricted to only one plane that of the long axis of the nerve from which they arise.

Types

- Localised

Table 1 Types of neurofibroma.		
	Diffuse	**Plexiform**
Common sites	Typically head and neck region	• Craniofacial 35% • Limbs 19%
Pathology	Low malignant transformation rate	Most growth in the first decade of life. Has a risk of malignant transformation
Genetic type	Sporadic or associated with NF1	Congenital related to NF1
Presentation	Ill-defined nodular lesion involving skin and subcutaneous tissue	Large tumours attached to major nerves. Serpentine or 'Bag of worms' under the skin
Surgery	Excision but has a potential to recur	Excision but has a high recurrence rate

NF1, neurofibromatosis type 1.

- Diffuse
- Plexiform

Multiple neurofibromatosis type 1 (NF1) is a congenital genetically transmitted condition that should be suspected if greater than 6 *café-au-lait spots* are present. It is quite common for children to have one or two spots but six or more must raise the suspicion of NF1.

NF1 or *Von Recklinghausen's disease* presents with:

- Cafe-au-lait spots
- Freckling
- Optic gliomas

NF2 or neurofibromatosis 2 (schwannomatosis) is a rare genetic condition where non-cancerous tumours grow in the brain, inner ear or spinal cord. Tumours such as acoustic neuroma (vestibular schwannomas) affect hearing and balance.

Lymph nodes

The subcutaneous nodes are in areas where there is nodal drainage, such as axilla, supraclavicular fossa, and groins. When noted the area that is draining to these nodes must also be examined for inflammation or malignancy.

Areas of drainage:

- Head and neck drains to cervical nodes
- Supra clavicular nodes drain the thorax and abdomen via thoracic duct on the left. Left supraclavicular node (Virchow's node) drains gastric and intra-abdominal malignancy
- Breast drains to the axillary nodes
- Testes drains to the para-aortic nodes (NOT inguinal)
- Below umbilicus drainage is to the inguinal nodes
- Tonsils drains to the jugulodigastric node
- Rings of Waldeyer

- Superficial Waldeyer's ring is a ring of lymphoid tissue at the naso- and oropharynx formed by the pharyngeal (adenoid), palatine, and lingual tonsils, acting as the first immune barrier to inhaled and ingested pathogens.
- Deep Waldeyer's ring is formed by the upper deep cervical lymph nodes.
- The superficial ring provides primary immune defense, while the deep ring provides lymphatic drainage and secondary immune response.

Inspection and palpation of subcutaneous lumps

It is advantageous to follow a protocol when examining these lumps. This is referred to as the 6 Ss and helps to define the lumps clearly.

1. *S*ite
2. *S*ize
3. *S*hape
4. *S*kin overlying the lump – healthy, colour – red and dusky
5. *S*urface – smooth, bosselated and engorged veins
6. *S*urrounding area/structures – increased vascularity

An organised examination and thought process is not only impressive, but it also reflects an organised mind with a sound approach.

Palpation helps to define the nature of the pathology.

- Acute
- Inflammatory
- Indolent

This assists in planning the management. If it is warm and tender, it signifies inflammation. A long-standing lipoma with no recent change in size may be well left alone after discussion with the patient. In other cases, removal may be necessary from the symptomatic or diagnostic point of view as when a histology may be needed to confirm the nature of the pathology.

Other benign lesions of the skin:

- Naevus
- Seborrhoeic warts are benign, pigmented, "stuck-on" epidermal tumours of the elderly with no malignant potential.
- Haemangioma is a benign vascular tumour caused by proliferation of blood vessels, commonly seen in infancy and childhood
- Arteriovenous fistula is a direct artery-to-vein communication causing a pulsatile, bruit-associated swelling that may lead to high-output cardiac failure. These could be congenital or traumatic.

Naevus

A naevus is a benign proliferation of melanocyte. This can be congenital or acquired.

Congenital naevi are of many different types. 'Café-au-lait' spots are commonly seen in fair skinned persons.

Naevi are classified depending on the site of location within the skin.

- *Dermal naevi* are a collection of naevus cell nests in the dermis

- *Junctional naevi* are nests at the junction of dermis and epidermis
- *Compound naevi* have naevus nests in the epidermis as well as in the dermis

Dermatoscopy has given rise to newer classifications

Sun exposure may lead to the formation of naevi.

Some acquired naevi involute with time and others may fade.

Currently, the preferred management is a referral to a dermatologist for management rather surgical removal.

Melanoma of the skin

This malignant tumour of the skin arises from melanocytes. About 30% of them arise from pre-existing moles. The most common risk factor is exposure to the sun. Many are pigmented and look black or brown. Some rare ones can be amelanotic.

The early recognition and management are now carried out by dermatologists in some countries, like the UK. A pigmented lesion can be a melanoma and suspicion is assessed with the ABCDE, guidance of the American Association of Dermatologists:

- *A*symmetry: The two halves do not match
- *B*order: Edges are not smooth
- *C*olour: Mottled and uneven, with shades of brown, black, white and pink
- *D*iameter: The spot is greater than the tip of a pencil eraser (6.0 mm)
- *E*volving: New lesion or change in size, shape, or colour.

Management

Early lesions are removed under local anaesthesia by the 'office dermatologist'.

The staging is based on the TNM system, but Clark's and Breslow's staging (**Tables 2 and 3**) are also used to prognosticate.

Table 2 Clark's staging is based on the pathological depth of invasion.

Level 1	In situ lesion in epidermis
Level 2	Superficial dermis
Level 3	Deep dermis
Level 4	Reticular dermis
Level 5	Subcutaneous tissue

Table 3 Breslow's staging is based on the numerical depth and correlates strongly with survival. The more superficial the lesion the better the survival.

Level 1	Up to 0.75 mm
Level 2	0.76–1.5 mm
Level 3	1.51–4 mm
Level 4	>4 mm

Types of melanomas

- *Superficial spreading melanoma:* It is the most common type of melanoma. It occurs more commonly in the fair-skinned persons. It is usually flat and superficial as the name indicates. The edges are irregular with variegated colour of different shades of black and brown.
- *Nodular melanoma:* These are typically modules that grow into the deeper layers. They tend to occur mostly in the torso and limbs
- *Lentigo maligna melanoma:* These melanomas develop in *Hutchinson's melanotic freckle.* These are found in areas exposed to the sun such as face and neck.
- *Amelanotic melanoma*
- *Acral lentiginous melanoma* occurs in the palm and sole of the feet. *Subungual melanoma* is a subtype that occurs as a pigmented lesion in the nail and can be mistaken for a haematoma.

Surgical intervention is needed for:

- Sentinel node biopsy when the lesion is larger than 8 mm
- Lymphadenectomy when regional nodes are involved
- Lymph node clearance
- Metastasectomy

Squamous cell carcinoma

These present in areas of the body exposed to sunlight. They are seldom life-threatening. They also occur in parts of the body that are not exposed to sunlight such as in the anal canal suggesting the presence of causes other than exposure to ultraviolet (UV) rays.

It often presents as an ulcer or a new skin lesion. They may also arise in old scars when it is referred to as a *Marjolin's ulcer*. Like all cancers they tend to spread in contiguity to the deeper layers and to the regional lymph nodes. When recognised early and confirmed histologically they can be treated by:

- Curettage and electrodessication of the base for small cancers
- Mohs surgery after Frederick Mohs. This is a laborious microscopic clearance layer by layer until malignancy is cleared. The procedure is applicable in parts of the body where skin is at a premium such as around the eyes, nose, etc. Elsewhere in the body, its value is questionable.
- Excision and primary closure

For advanced cancers as in common with other skin cancers the surgical treatment is directed towards wide *'tri-dimensional'* excision and clearance of regional nodes if they are involved. Skin grafts or rotation flaps may be needed if there is a large defect to bridge after excision.

Basal cell carcinoma

The most common skin cancers arising from basal cells of the epidermis. The basal cells replenish dead cells. The DNA of these cells are susceptible to mutations when exposed to *UV rays.* They occur as tiny transparent lesions or ulcers in parts of the body exposed to the sun like the face, ears, neck, etc. They are characterised by local invasion and destruction and seldom if ever metastasise. *Ageing* and *immuno-suppression* are other factors. Much of the principles of treatment is similar to the management of early squamous cell cancers.

Burns

Types of burn:

- Thermal
- Electrical
- Radiation
- Chemical

Level of burn:

- *First degree:* This is also referred to as superficial burns. A scald is a typical example. The burn involves the most superficial layer. It is red and *painful but does not blister*
- *Second degree (partial thickness burns)*: This involves the epidermis and superficial dermis. It is red and *painful. Blister formation occurs*
- *Third degree (full thickness or deep burns):* This involves the deeper dermis and subcutaneous tissue. The nerves and blood vessels are destroyed and, therefore, *there is no pain,* and it looks grey and ashen

Assessment

As in assessment of any patient, the immediate management is directed towards *A*irway, *B*reathing, *C*irculation, *D*isability and *E*xposure for examination.

Primary goal is *airway* and *fluid management* for serious burns. This is directed towards assessing the *total body surface area* affected by the burn and stabilising the patient.

With *electrical burn,* one must be aware of the possibility of *cardiac* and *proximal vessel injury* or even necrosis leading to more major complications than first recognised at presentation. For instance, an electrical burn to the hand may lead to loss of viability of the whole upper limb with the patient needing proximal amputation as the author has seen.

Extent of the burn

- Percentage of body surface involved – rule of nine; this assists in the fluid management and plan provision of skin cover to prevent fluid loss and sepsis
- Injury to airways

The depth and percentage of body surface that is affected has an impact not only on the level of care a patient is likely to need immediately but also the prognosis and complications. Smoke inhalation and injury to airways need immediate assessment. *Singeing of vibrissae* must alert one to the possibility of thermal lung injury.

Rule of nine (Table 4)

This is a useful formula to calculate the extent of percentage of total body surface area (TBSA) burnt.

Treatment

The aim of immediate resuscitation in a severely burned patient is to ensure good perfusion of the organs with the aim of preventing organ failure.

Table 4 Rule of nine for total body surface area (TBSA) burnt.	
Part of the body	**Body surface area**
Head and neck	9%
Each upper limb	9% times 2 = 18%
Each lower limb	18% times 2 = 36%
Anterior torso	18%
Posterior torso	18%
Perineum	1%

This translates to intravenous fluids and monitoring of urine output. *Where facilities permit patients with >25% TBSA burn are best treated in an HDU with monitoring.*

Fluids

Crystalloids can be used for fluid resuscitation and the amount needed is calculated as per the *'Parkland formula'* that is commonly used for fluid replacement in the first 24 hours. This formula has improved outcomes in the management of children with 10% BSB and in adults with 20% BSB.

Parkland formula seeks to infuse fluids at:

- *4 mL/kg bodyweight per percent of TBSA burn in the first 24 hours*
- Half of the calculated volume is infused in the first 8 hours
- The rest of the fluid in the next 16 hours

The total quantity if calculated to be >6 mL/kg then albumin replacement should be considered lest the over infusion of crystalloids leads to complications such as:

- Compartment syndrome of extremities/abdomen
- Cerebral oedema
- Adult respiratory distress syndrome (ARDS)
- Multiple organ dysfunction

The term *'fluid creep'* was coined by Pruitt in 2000 when resuscitation volumes were in excess leading to the possibility of above complications.

Under infusion can lead to renal failure and MODS.

Catheterisation

Since there can be harm from both over and under infusion of fluids, it is best to aim for a urine output of 30–50 mL/h.

Prevention of stress ulcers – Curling's ulcer

When the percentage of burn is >20% then the possibility of gastric ulceration increases. This is thought to be due to a reduction in splanchnic perfusion leading to reduced gastric blood supply causing atrophy and ulceration. It can be prevented by usage of proton pump inhibitors and an awareness of the possibility of *gastric dilatation* when patient complains of epigastric pain. This can be treated with nasogastric tube insertion.

For burn patients, presence of epigastric pain and major burn with TBSA > 20% showed significant association with ulcer development (Young Hwan Choi).

Subsequent treatment is undertaken by the plastic surgeons. The treatment is geared towards:

- Control of pain
- Prevention of infection
- Provision of skin cover

Prevention of infection: In major burns, this is most important as it can lead to sepsis rapidly. Antibiotic cover and dressing of the skin should go hand in hand with fluid resuscitation. Various types of antiseptic dressings are available, but they differ in their ability in preventing the formation of eschar.

Topical dressings include:

- Silver sulfadiazine
- Silver nitrate solution
- Silver-impregnated dressings
- Mafenide acetate ointment
- Bacitracin ointment
- Polymyxin ointment
- Myostatin ointment (nystatin – anti-fungal)

The burn is dressed loosely with gauze impregnated with any of the above-mentioned medicines.

The most common infective agent is *Staphylococcus* and the dreaded MRSA *infection.* These can lead to burn sepsis.

It goes without saying the *sepsis protocol* must be introduced at the earliest opportunity if a focus of infection is identified.

In second-degree burns, if blisters are noted they *must not be aspirated for fear of introduction of infection.*

Most patients with major burns require referral to a major burn centre with experience in management of these seriously ill patients.

Provision of early skin cover after the necessary debridement in serious burns enables better outcomes.

Allograft and *autografts* are used in combination where sufficient skin cover is not possible.

Chapter 13

General paediatric surgery

Srinivasan Ravi

Definition of general paediatric surgery

This aspect of paediatric surgery addresses common problems in paediatric surgery that are dealt with by a non-specialist general surgeon. The management covers:

- Phimosis
- Hernia
- Undescended testes
- Hydrocoele
- Appendicitis
- Skin lesions

Phimosis

This is one of the common conditions that is seen in a general paediatric service. Phimosis is the name given when the foreskin that covers the glans penis cannot be fully retracted. This is *more often a physiological problem* than a pathological problem. As the child grows, the foreskin will usually become fully retractile without need for surgical intervention.

The reason why circumcision became common practice in some countries such as the USA is because of concepts in the Middle East. Among the Jews circumcision is practised soon after birth on the 8th day. This required the excision of the whole of the foreskin. In the Middle East and in sub-Saharan Africa, a partial excision of the foreskin or division of the frenulum alone is practised. The proponents of circumcision claim that it reduces the risk of penile cancers as well as HIV (foreskin is rich in HIV target cells McCoombe & Short - 2006). A review of three randomised control studies in sub-Saharan Africa has found that in areas where there is high prevalence of circumcision there is indeed a reduction in the rates of cancers of the penis along with reduction in HIV and sexually transmitted disease. High-quality evidence suggests that there is evidence of less harm when a circumcision is carried out properly under expert care. There is also very little evidence of long-standing harm. There was also reduction in the risk of *human papilloma virus* in those who underwent circumcision as well as in their partners once again probably relating to the absence of injury (micro tears) during insertive intercourse.

Phimosis may present as:

- *Balanitis* which is inflammation of the glans penis
- *Balanoposthitis* which is inflammation of the glands and the prepuce

- *Paraphimosis*
- *Urinary infection*

In most cases, balanitis and balanoposthitis settle spontaneously without intervention.

Paraphimosis occurs when the foreskin following retraction is not fully or only partially reduced. The foreskin then becomes oedematous, painful, and subsequently difficult to reduce. In most cases, reduction can be achieved by compression to relieve the oedema along with gentle traction. Following even a single such episode, the children merit a circumcision.

Urinary tract infection is less common but can occur because of a tight phimosis. In these situations, residual urine tends to collect in the preputial sack. Longstanding irritation due to chemical changes in the residual urine can cause ammoniacal dermatitis leading to further exacerbation of preputial inflammation leading to in some cases infection (posthitis).

Surgery for circumcision is a relatively straightforward procedure and under ideal conditions carries very little complications. In the US, nearly 60% of male children are circumcised soon after birth. In the UK, circumcision is avoided as a routine practice and implemented only in the presence of complications of phimosis. The surgery is deferred until the child is older and the patients are advised not to retract the foreskin and to dab the urine at the end of micturition.

In sub-Saharan Africa, circumcision is a commonly carried out procedure but there are no true statistics available.

The two major complications are:

1. Bleeding
2. Infection

Neither of these is likely to have longstanding or serious complications.

Hernia

- Inguinal and umbilical hernia
- In infants and children, inguinal hernia and umbilical herniae are not uncommon. Inguinal hernia is more common in male babies.

Embryology

*Key points in the descent of the testis (**Figure 1**)*

- Testis develops as an intra-abdominal organ in the mesonephric ridge alongside the embryologic kidney
- It subsequently migrates to its final location in the scrotum guided by the *gubernaculum*
- The gubernaculum is a fibrous cord that is attached to the developing testis at one end and to the scrotum at the other
- The rigid gubernaculum by not growing along at the same rate as the growing embryo pulls the testis down to the scrotum
- If the gubernaculum is attached to the scrotum, then the descent of the testis occurs as per expectations
- If the dissent of the test is impeded along its expected line of descent due to either a fat pad at the external ring of the inguinal canal or due to *short blood vessels* as is more common, then the testis is referred to as an *undescended testis*

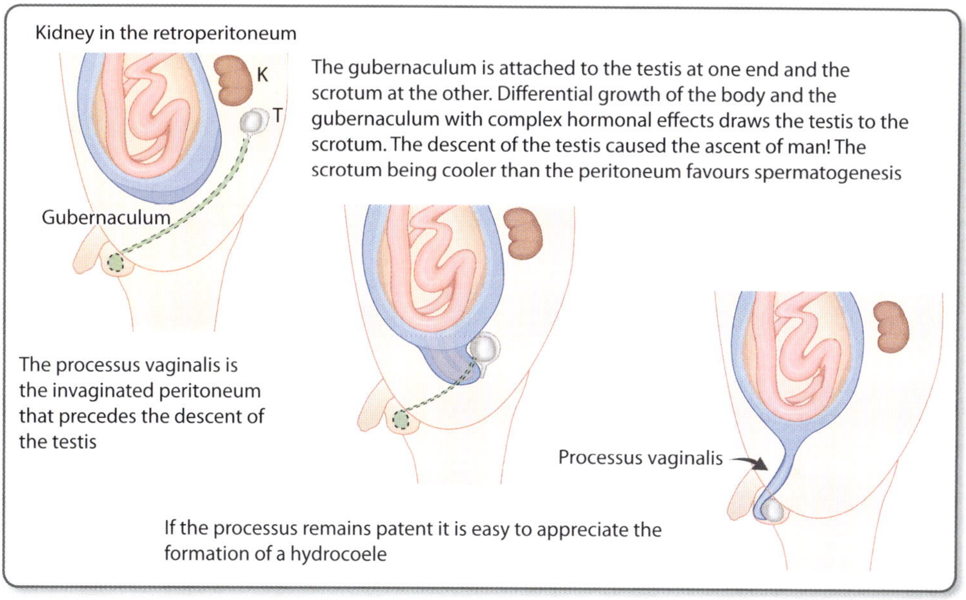

Figure 1 The descent of the testis.

- If the gubernaculum is attached elsewhere such as to the groin or to the perineum (a paper on the gubernacular tails, by Lockwood, 1888), the testis may be located at places other than its natural final position and is referred to as an *ectopic testis*. The current biological evidence suggests a more complex process and no longer supports the gubernacular tails of Lockwood. It is, however, easy to understand the various locations of an ectopic testis
- In certain cases, the testis is located along its line of descent but tends to pull up into the groin in the inguinal canal but there appears to be no impediment to its final descent and this is called a *retractile testis*

As the testis descends along its path it pulls a layer of the peritoneum in front of it which is referred to as the *processus vaginalis testis*. In the normal course of events once the testis reaches its scrotal position the processus vaginalis closes behind it.

In a small proportion of babies, the processus remains open allowing fluid from the peritoneum to collect in the enveloping layers of the testis forming a *hydrocoele*.

Most of these the hydrocoeles settle spontaneously by the age of two without recourse to surgery.

In a small proportion of children, a surgical intervention is necessary. *More importantly, if it is present at birth a distinction must be made between a hernia and a hydrocoele.*

This distinction may be difficult clinically. Ultrasound scan may help to clarify the diagnosis by noting the presence of bowel loops within the sac.

If a hernia is detected urgent surgical intervention is necessary as the risk of strangulation is high in babies.

It must, of course, be noted that in the infants the inguinal canal is not fully developed, and the internal and external rings are in apposition and not oblique. Consequently, majority of the herniae that appear to be irreducible do reduce spontaneously but occasionally it can lead to strangulation and, hence, the urgency to remedy it surgically.

Umbilicus and umbilical hernia

Umbilicus is a cicatrix that is left behind after the umbilical cord falls away. It contains umbilical arteries as well as digestive and urological structures. Embryologically, it is an important point of confluence in the abdominal wall.

This area becomes more important as it is involved in the rotation of the bowel. The volume of the developing peritoneal cavity is quite restricted and it is, therefore, unable to accommodate the growing loops of small bowel accompanied by the rotation that occurs along with the growth. The small bowel extrudes into the umbilical cord that is attached to the placenta and within it there occurs a *rotation of 180°* in the *anticlockwise* direction. The bowel then returns to the peritoneal cavity, all at the umbilicus. The umbilicus then closes very much like a shutter in a camera. The circumference of the umbilicus contracts leaving a cicatrix. When this mechanism fails or is incomplete a hernia occurs. This is a *true umbilical hernia* as it occurs in the main defect in the umbilicus. As opposed to this, in adults, it occurs alongside the original cicatrix in the presence of an acquired defect. In most children, the umbilical shutter closes by the age of 3 leaving a reasonably intact wall. The need for surgical correction of the umbilical hernia in children in the early stages needs very careful consideration. *It is now a common practice to undertake repair only after the age of 3.* It may be necessary earlier if the hernia progress in size.

In certain other situations, the anterior abdominal wall may fail to close leaving a split from the umbilicus proximally to varying distance up to the xiphisternum. There are three types of defects.

1. *Exomphalos minor:* The defect is minor, and the contents are enveloped in a membranous sac. In most cases, the defect can be closed without any major problem.
2. *Exomphalos major:* The defect is larger than the minor exomphalos. *The bowel is enveloped in a sac* and sometimes contains organs along with the bowel. This will need a more complicated operation but, in most of the patients, provision of skin cover will be possible. It may, however, need to be staged to get adequate muscular approximation. *There may be associated genetic defects.*
3. *Gastroschisis:* In this situation, there is *no sac* and bowel is open to the exterior. Immediate skin cover is not possible. The repair is achieved by enveloping the bowel in a plastic sack called a 'silo'. This is like that of a freezer bag or a balloon and envelopes all of the bowel. The bag is then tightened gradually from the top pushing the bowel into the abdominal cavity over a period of time. Staged repair will in most cases fully approximate the abdominal wall.

Exomphalos or omphalocoele differs from gastroschisis by the presence of a membranous sac which is absent in the latter.

Chapter 14

Perioperative care

Srinivasan Ravi

Introduction

Length of stay (LOS) (**Figure 1**) in hospital is a surrogate marker for comorbidities, complications and quality of care. Postoperative complications are not uncommon. Its early recognition and correction reflect the quality of care that is delivered. Intraoperative complications and delayed recognition of postoperative complications increase morbidity, prolong in patient stay and may lead to mortality.

Recognising the surgical risk is challenging and used to be wholly subjective. With accumulation of large amounts of data in the UK by the National Confidential Enquiry into Patient Outcome and Death (NCEPOD) (**Table 1**) we are now able to offer a more realistic prediction of the risk of morbidity and mortality following any surgical intervention. Stratifying the risk prior to emergency surgical intervention permits an assessment of the risk versus benefits of that intervention for that individual patient. The risk of mortality and major complications after surgery in the total general surgical population is <1% of all patients undergoing an operation (Knowing the risk – NCEPOD). In patients older than 80 years of age, the morbidity and mortality rate rises with increasing age. The most common comorbidity in that age group was hypertension and dyspnoea as noted in one study on surgical risk factors, morbidity and mortality in

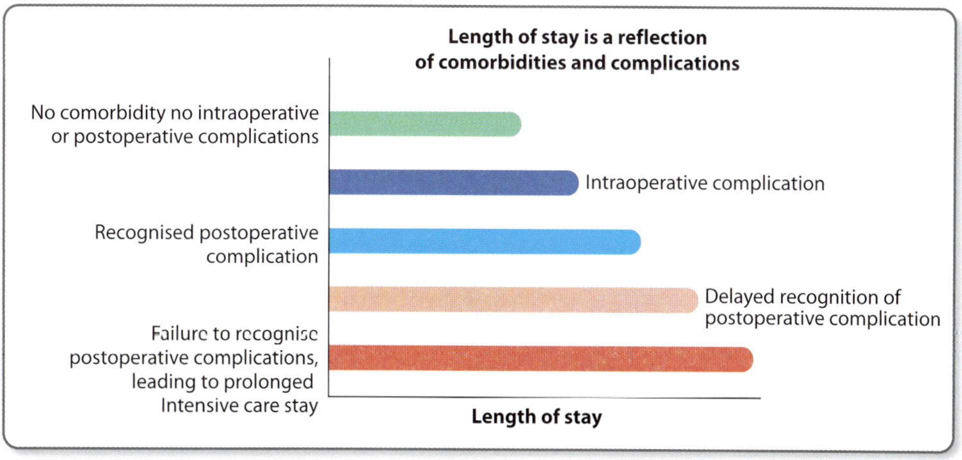

Figure 1 Length of stay (LOS) in a hospital.

Table 1 NCEPOD (National Confidential Enquiry into Patient Outcome and Death, UK) classification of surgical urgency of intervention.

Level of urgency	Time to action
Immediate	Within minutes – threat to life, limb, organ
Urgent	Within hours – perforated viscus following resuscitation
Expedited	Within days – diverticulitis without perforation
Elective	Within months – planned with the patient. Hernia repair
Risk of surgical morbidity and mortality increases with the level of urgency	

elderly patients. In this study, the morbidity rate and mortality rates rose with increasing age, with a morbidity of 51% and a mortality rate of 7% in patients older than 80 years of age. *Furthermore, in the over 80 years old patients, a 30-minute increase in operative duration increased the odds of mortality by 17%.*

In this study, age was statistically significantly associated with morbidity and mortality as was emergency operations, preoperative impairment of activities of daily living and ASA scores across all age groups.

In another study assessing the impact of *intraoperative complications, (Intraoperative Adverse Events in Abdominal Surgery: What Happens in the Operating Room Does Not Stay in the Operating Room)* a total of 9,288 cases were studied; 183 had intraoperative adverse events (iAEs) causing bowel (44%) or vessel (29%) injuries intraoperatively. iAEs were independently associated with substantial and significant increases in postoperative mortality, morbidity, and prolonged LOS.

Postoperative complications associated with iAEs included:

- Deep/organ-space surgical site infection
- Sepsis
- Pneumonia
- Failure to wean

Morbidity and mortality

Morbidity refers to illness or disease. Comorbidity is the disease that is associated with another disease. For example, hypertension and cardiovascular disease, hepatitis and hepatocellular carcinoma, obesity and diabetes.

Mortality is death and mortality rates are deaths from different diseases. Morbidity and mortality rates increase with the following factors:

- Comorbidity
- Age
- Level of urgency
- Duration of surgery

Surgical outcome risk

The outcome of surgery can be predicted (to a certain extent) with respect to the degree of postoperative morbidity that a particular surgical intervention may cause. The percentage of mortality can also be similarly predicted. There are various tools available for this. This type of prediction is a valuable tool for discussions with carers, critical care team and anaesthetists.

The prerequisites of diligent care involve:

- Preoperative evaluation in elective cases
- Reducing intraoperative complications
- Early recognition of postoperative complications
- Daily ward rounds
- Tracking of the NEWS scores
- Triggering a response as appropriate
- Reviewing the results of investigations
- Reviewing medications
- Clear, dated and signed documentation
- Good hand over at the end of a shift
- Clear and unambiguous communication with patients and when needed, with the carers or relatives

Postoperative pain control

Focussing on pain control as part of the primary assessment separately will define its importance. ABCDE-P should be the norm even though pain is expected to be assessed as part of the ABCDE assessment.

In the postoperative period, provision of adequate pain control is paramount in enabling mobilisation and deep breathing. Pain is detrimental to postoperative progress. It may be a manifestation of prolonged surgery and implementation of poor pain control.

The consequences of pain, especially after laparotomy, may initially only affect the respiratory system but soon the cardiovascular system will be affected. Pain causes tachycardia and *tachycardia tires the heart!* Cardiac perfusion is best during the diastolic phase. With tachycardia, diastole is shortened with serious consequences to perfusion of the heart, especially in the elderly.

The most obvious manifestation of postoperative abdominal pain is shallow breathing. *Shallow breathing* leads to restricted pulmonary movements. This leads to *'dead space air ventilation'* which is richer in carbon dioxide than freshly inhaled air. It is not just the rate that matters but also the depth of respiration. Deeper the breathing, greater the oxygenation. Increased rate of respiration may yet lead to hypoxia due to dead space air ventilation. Breathing dead space air lowers the FiO_2 and can lead to hypoxia. The shallow breathing can also lead to *atelectasis* and in some elderly patients to subsequent *pneumonia, sepsis* and *cardiac failure.*

Opiates are the queen of analgesics and need to be used appropriately to enable *early physiotherapy and mobilisation.* These lead to improved chest movement and better lung function. Respiratory rate in the postoperative period may well be a marker of poor analgesia as much as acidosis.

Physiology of pain

Pain is a protective mechanism that allows the organism to withdraw from danger or damage inducing objects. Factors that enhance pain include the emotional status of the patient and, hence, dealing with pain requires a great degree of sensitivity. The pain and touch points in the body were mapped out in the 19th century. The pressure required to cause the *pin-prick sensation* was noted to be different from that required to cause *touch.* It was subsequently shown that *two types of nerve fibres transmit pain to the brain.* The damaged skin transmits pain through *thin C fibres* that are not medullated. They reach the posterior horn where there are fast firing *A-β fibres* that are medullated and transmit non-pain signals. *Melzack and Wall* in the 1960s showed that by stimulating the A-β fibres, the transmission of pain signals can be blocked. This is the mechanism by which 'rubbing it better' works. By rubbing the skin, the A-β fibres are activated and block transmission of the signals from the C fibres. Acupuncture may also be explained by a similar mechanism.

Pain can be controlled by many ways.

- *Centrally* by opiates and analgesics
- *Neuraxially* by spinal and epidurals
- *Paraxially* by various blocks
- *Peripherally* by local anaesthetic agents

Opiates

Opiates are derivatives of opium. *Morphine* is the queen of analgesics. There are many types of opiates, but the commonly used ones are morphine and *Codeine. Fentanyl and heroin* are other types in use for sedation and analgesia.

The opiates act agonistically on specific receptors called μ, δ, and κ. These, in turn, stimulate the *g-proteins* on the cell membrane leading to change in configuration and internal messaging. This inhibits the neurons in the dorsal horn and blocks pain signals from the periphery. They also activate midbrain areas (periaqueductal grey) and send signals (descending inhibition) to inhibit pain transmission. Morphine and derivatives act on μ-receptors present in the *dorsal horn of the spinal cord,* central nervous system especially in areas related to pain such as *thalamus* and *periaqueductal grey.* These receptors are also found in the *respiratory system and gastrointestinal system* (hence, respiratory depression and constipation are side effects of morphine). Codeine, though less effective than morphine, is less addictive and is more commonly used.

In the postoperative period, morphine can be prescribed as a PCA or patient-controlled analgesia. This is possible only when the patient has *capacity* and does not have any mechanical problems such as arthritis or neurological deficits that restrict movements of the limbs. It is very useful in patients who can understand the principles of PCA. Language may thus be a barrier.

Prescription writing for these drugs is very stringent requiring the dosage to be written in words as well as in numbers. Always refer to the national formulary prior to writing it and follow the protocols required for the respective country.

Paracetamol

Reduces pain and pyrexia but not inflammation. Mechanism of action is unclear. Pain is due to the production of prostaglandins following injury. Prostaglandins potentiate pain that is caused by inflammatory mediators such as histamine and bradykinin. They sensitise the nerve endings and manifest as pain. It is believed that paracetamol must act in some way to decrease the effect of prostaglandins possibly by suppressing COX2. The mechanism of action may be a combination of central and peripheral effects. The NNT for pain control with paracetamol is 1.7.

Nonsteroidal anti-inflammatory drugs

This group of drugs includes *aspirin, ibuprofen and diclofenac sodium*. Interestingly, the NNT for pain control with this group of drugs is 1 suggesting that it is better at controlling pain than paracetamol.

They are classified into *nonselective* and *selective* nonsteroidal anti-inflammatory drugs (NSAIDs) based on their action on *cyclo-oxygenase* (COX). They reversibly inhibit these enzymes unlike aspirin which irreversibly inhibits the enzyme thus affecting platelets for their lifetime of 8–9 days. This is the reason that aspirin effects take a week to be abolished.

COX1: This enzyme has a physiological protective function on *gastric and intestinal epithelium, renal* and *platelet aggregation* function. Thromboxane A2 is synthesised in platelets through COX1 enzyme activity causing vaso-constriction and platelet aggregation. Aspirin inhibits this irreversibly, *reducing platelet aggregation and production.* The inhibition of the protective effect of COX1 on gastric and renal function is the reason for their side effects on gastric and renal function.

COX2: It is unexpressed normally but it is driven by inflammation and is referred to as *inflammatory prostaglandin.*

Inhibition of COX1 and -2 in a non-selective or selective way provides relief from pain. Selective COX2 inhibitors do not cause gastric symptoms but their side effects include cardiac and CVA-related problems.

Gabapentin

This is an anti-convulsant which also benefits neuropathic pain such as postherpetic pain. In 2018, a meta-analysis showed that it was of no benefit for sciatica but benefited the spasticity of multiple sclerosis. It must be appreciated that *gabapentin is not an analgesic in the routine sense of the term.*

Patient-controlled analgesia (PCA)

When a patient controls the amount of analgesia needed, it is more effective than non-PCA. (Pastino A, Lakra A. Patient-Controlled Analgesia).

PCA can be instilled through:

- Central lines
- Peripheral veins
- Epidural lines
- Through skin, i.e. fentanyl patch with a button to press

The system was introduced in the 1970s but has evolved to different types of pumps to deliver the medication through the various lines.

The main components are:

- Patient-controlled button – for self-delivery
- A mechanical pump

- Medication chamber – containing either opiate alone or opiate and a local anaesthetic, normally, bupivacaine
- Programming screen – for minimum effective dose to be run in the background with lock out period
- Locking device – to prevent overdosing by the patient or by proxy by relatives

The contraindications to its use:
- Lack of capacity on the part of the patient
- Sedation
- Inability to comprehend the system – language barrier
- Inability to use the hand to manipulate the button, e.g. rheumatoid arthritis
- Allergy to medications
- Chronic renal failure, antithrombotic therapy, sleep apnoea and bleeding disorder

Local anaesthetic drugs

The most common agent is lignocaine, also called lidocaine and xylocaine.
- It has been in use since 1948
- It is the most used local anaesthetic throughout the world
- It *acts by inhibiting sodium channels* and when infiltrated close to nerves it closes the sodium channel and, thus, stops propagation of nerve conduction. In the heart, the same effect decreases the heart rate and, hence, it is useful in managing ventricular arrhythmias when amiodarone is contraindicated
- It acts more rapidly than bupivacaine
- Bupivacaine, however, is longer acting

Combining lignocaine with adrenaline:
- Reduces bleeding
- Doubles the duration of action due to the accompanying vasoconstriction leading to slower absorption
- Doubles the quantity that can be used from 3.5 mg/kg body weight to 7 mg/kg

Toxicity is manifest as central nervous system (CNS) and cardiovascular system (CVS) effects.
- *CNS:* Circumoral tingling and numbness, anxiety, agitation and seizures leading to confusion and coma
- *CVS:* Hypotension, bradycardia, arrhythmia, and cardiac arrest
- *Other side effects:* Tinnitus and urticaria

Management of toxicity starts with recognising that excess dosage has been instilled. This is followed by stopping the infusion of local anaesthesia (as in epidural analgesia) and giving immediate *intravenous lipid emulsion infusion.*

Other local anaesthetic drugs:
- *Bupivacaine hydrochloride:* Slow but longer action compared to others
- *Prilocaine hydrochloride:* Has a low toxicity

Epidural analgesia

According to the faculty of pain management of the Royal College of Anaesthetists, epidural anaesthesia is very effective in the management of postoperative pain.

- Continuous epidural analgesia has major implications and so *needs an informed consent*
- There must be 24-hour access to expert care and advice
- Anticoagulant usage is discontinued well prior to inserting epidural, during insertion and removal. It is avoided while epidural is in use as it can lead to complications of haematoma in the epidural space and worse, paralysis
- Aseptic principles apply from the time of insertion to removal
- Some degree of sensory block may occur
- Monitoring complications while the epidural is in use will promote early action
- *Complications:*
  - Infection
  - Abscess
  - Haematoma
  - Hypotension: Other postoperative causes such as bleeding and myocardial infarction need to be excluded
  - Respiratory suppression and drowsiness if opiates are used. These effects can be reversed with medications like naloxone
  - Postepidural headache
  - Increasing motor blockage (Bromage scale)
  - Urinary retention
  - Pruritus, if opiate is used
  - Neuropraxia or nerve damage
  - Total spinal is a sinister complication with respiratory arrest and cardiovascular collapse. The patient will need supportive therapy in the ITU
  - Failure of analgesia

Bromage scale scores the degree of block:

1. Complete paralysis
2. Foot movement alone
3. Foot and just able to flex knee
4. Full range of movement

When there is complete paralysis overdosage or pressure effect due to haematoma or abscess must be suspected.

Epidural infusion

- Epidural infusion bags will need replacing every 24 hours even if not fully used
- The epidural catheter is removed in 3–4 days to prevent the risk of infection and sepsis
- Aseptic care must be always provided and also at times of manipulation of kinks or disconnections
- *The infusate can be:*
  - *Standard infusion* with fentanyl 2 µg/mL in 250 mL of 0.1% bupivacaine
  - *Opiate-free infusion* – 250 mL of 0.125% bupivacaine

The infusion rate can be titrated to control pain. It will vary from 2 to 15 mL/h.

Respiratory rate must be monitored as *excess dosage will suppress respiration.*

Rectus sheath catheter

- This avoids complications of epidural anaesthesia as the effect provided is limited to the abdominal wall
- There are very few systemic effects other than those related to the local anaesthetic infiltration
- The procedure is carried out under vision prior to closing the abdomen
- The catheter is inserted posterior to the rectus muscle but anterior to the posterior sheath
- This plane is easy to access during the first laparotomy
- Finding this plane in re-operations may be difficult

Infusate

Normally 400 mL of 0.125% bupivacaine is infused at the rate of 10 mL/h.

Transabdominal plane block

- This block is instilled in the anterolateral abdominal wall in the intermuscular plane between the internal oblique and the transversus abdominis
- When instilled under ultrasound guidance in the correct plane, it blocks the dermatomes (T6 to L1) of the mid and lower abdomen from the midline to the mid-clavicular line
- It is effective for up to 24 hours
- Instillation is done at the time of surgery

Oxygen

Oxygen should be treated as a drug. It is perhaps the most common drug that is used in surgical emergencies. It should certainly be one of the first drugs in sepsis and shock. In most acutely ill patients, the arterial carbon dioxide, the $PaCO_2$ is either normal or low. Maintaining an oxygen saturation of 94–98% is desirable.

The delivery of oxygen can be:

- *High concentration oxygen* therapy (high flow) as is used in patients with sepsis, pneumonia, hypotension, and anaphylaxis. In these patients, there is little risk of CO_2 retention. The respiratory rate is high. Both the oxygen and CO_2 levels are likely to be low. The oxygen saturation target is above *94% saturation.*
- *Low-concentration oxygen* as is used in patients with COPD. The oxygen delivery is targeted with a Venturi mask providing 24 or 28% concentration oxygen to maintain the saturation between *88 and 92%.*

The modes of delivery are discussed in Volume 1. Suffice it to say that commonly, they are delivered by:

- Nasal cannula
- Non-rebreathing mask

- Venturi mask
- Incubator
- CPAP – continuous positive airway pressure
- Intubation and ventilation

Hypoxia or low saturation may be noted when there is:
- Tachypnoea
- Dyspnoea
- Apnoea
- Tachycardia
- Hypotension
- Confusion and memory loss

Extracorporeal membrane oxygenation (ECMO): This is used in the intensive care in patients with cardiopulmonary complications of sepsis that fail to respond to various ventilatory manipulations. It can also be used as a bridge prior to cardiopulmonary transplant. The ECMO machine has a membrane oxygenator, which acts as an artificial lung and exchanges oxygen and carbon dioxide from blood
- *Venoarterial ECMO:* In this type of ECMO, the blood bypasses the heart completely. The blood is drawn out of a major vein and pumped back by the ECMO machine into a major artery
- *Venovenous ECMO:* This supports lungs alone when cardiac function is unaffected.

Chapter 15

Experiential case-based learning

Srinivasan Ravi

Experience both personal and transmitted over generations is a great teacher. I am going to discuss a few cases that transmit the experience to trainees. These are historic cases that are fully anonymised, enhanced and modified for learning. Some predate the implementation of modern-day investigations. There are a few basic principles that stand out in the management of surgical patients both in acute and elective situations.

P points:

- *P*atient first, *P*art next
  - Always examine the patient as a whole before concentrating on the part in question. Follow the rules of assessing physiology
- *P*hysiology before *P*athology
  - It is best to get the physiology right and stabilise the patient before any major surgical intervention
  - Sometimes it may have to be addressed simultaneously rather than in tandem
  - Abnormal pathology causes abnormal physiology
- *P*ulmonary and *P*ump (cardiac) functions are tightly linked
  - If the pump is affected, the pulmonary function will soon be affected
  - If the pulmonary function is affected the pump function deteriorates rapidly
- *P*oor pump function is mirrored by a poor renal function
  - If the *urine output* is low in the acute surgical situation the cardiac output will be low

1. *Shrapnel injury to the brachial artery. Patient first!*
   A 28-year-old man was struck in the left inner arm by a shrapnel during the first Iraq war of 1991. He presented to an orthopaedic surgeon a few days later. There was a tiny skin wound in the medial aspect of the left arm overlying the brachial artery. The orthopaedic surgeon following a brief examination concluded that this was an abscess. No neurological assessment was carried out. This patient was taken to the theatre and under general anaesthesia the 'abscess' was incised. To his horror, arterial blood spurted out. I was in the next theatre and was called to address this immediately. It became apparent that this was not an abscess but a pseudoaneurysm of the brachial artery secondary to a shrapnel injury. This is a classical presentation and I had only heard about it in textbooks. After a quick examination on the table, the incision was extended in the line of the brachial artery and rapid control of proximal and distal artery was obtained. A graft achieved good distal flow with palpable radial pulses.

During the operation the median nerve was injured and was reconstituted.

- Shrapnel injury or any injury with a sharp object over a major vessel can present as a hot tender read mass
- A similar situation pertains in IV drug users over the femoral vessels and following cardiac angiography
- It can often be mistaken for an abscess
- A pseudoaneurysm always needs to be excluded in any lump that overlies major vessels and also following injury during access.
- An ultrasound scan would have made the diagnosis and permitted better planning
- *Investigate before intervention* is a sound policy
- The median nerve is in close proximity to the vessels in the mid-arm. Deliberate dissection will avoid injury although in an emergency it may be injured. Distortion of the anatomy by the pseudoaneurysm could have contributed to the nerve being accidentally divided.

2. *Lucid interval in a 'head injury' patient treated as an alcoholic. 'Patient first' principle includes a clear history.*

   In 1984, A 36-year-old man accidentally fell and hit his head on the curb while walking in front of a 'pub'. An ambulance brought him to the accident and emergency (A&E) department when the patient who was semiconscious in the ambulance was noted to be awake and responding to questions. As he had been picked up in front of a pub it was presumed, he was drunk. When he was reviewed by the 'A&E' doctors later, he was comatose. The patient had not been drinking but had, in fact, fallen in front of a pub, sustaining a head injury. In the early 1980s, CT scan was not universally available. A mid-liner, an instrument that detected the shift of the midline showed a shift in the midline due to an extradural haemorrhage. Following a head injury, three types of intracranial pathology can occur.

   1. *Intracranial haemorrhage:* This can be extradural, subdural or intracranial
   2. A rise *in intracranial pressure due to oedema*
   3. A *midline shift:* Becker et al., in 1977, showed that a shift >1 cm could be fatal

   The period during which he was awake and stumbled into the ambulance is typical of a *lucid interval.*

   - Lucid interval can occur in patients with head injury
   - It is a temporary improvement in the conscious level of a patient following a head injury. It manifests as the intervening period of wakefulness between *initial loss of consciousness* due to *concussion* and subsequent loss of consciousness due to *increasing intracranial tension*
   - It is classical of extradural haemorrhage. Unlike subdural haemorrhage, which is normally venous, extradural haemorrhage is arterial and can lead to further loss of consciousness due to increasing intracranial pressure
   - *Monro-Kellie doctrine:* The skull is a rigid box containing three components:
     1. The brain
     2. The cerebrospinal fluid (CSF)
     3. The blood, mostly venous in the dural sinuses

   The doctrine states that if the volume of one of these components increases within the rigid cranium, then the intracranial pressure will rise. The intracranial pressure is normally maintained at 5–15 mm Hg because of an equilibrium between the components of the cranium. At a pressure of 20 mm Hg intervention may be needed to prevent life-threatening consequences.

The Cushing reflex: In 1901, Harvey Cushing noted that acute elevation of intracranial pressure (ICP) leads to a triad of physiological response. The triad consists of:

1. Widening of the pulse pressure (the gap between the systolic and diastolic pressures)
2. Bradycardia
3. Irregular respiration

Cushing also noted the occurrence of a gastric ulcer in patients with a head injury. It is now referred to as the Cushing Ulcer.

As the ICP increases the cerebral perfusion pressure (CPP) drops. CPP is the difference between the mean arterial pressure (MAP) and ICP. The normal CPP is between 70 and 80 mmHg.

Autoregulation of cerebral blood flow (CBF): The body maintains a constant CBF over a range of 50–150 mmHg of CPP. Beyond these limits a rise in CPP above 150 mmHg leads to dilatation of the cerebral blood vessels with consequent rise in cerebral blood volume and intracranial pressure. This can lead to cerebral oedema or cerebral haemorrhage. A fall in CPP below 50 mmHg leads to cerebral ischaemia.

3. *Anaemia in 'Meckel's diverticulum.' Chase the cause of the physiological abnormality.*
   In 1989, a 42-year-old man presented with a history of one episode of passing dark stools and a haemoglobin of 85 g/L. To exclude a gastrointestinal (GI) bleed, he had a gastroscopy and a colonoscopy both of which were normal. No diagnosis was made, and it was presumed that this was dietary. He was discharged without follow-up on oral iron. A year later the patient represented with a low haemoglobin. He again underwent a normal gastroscopy. This time, a Meckel's scan was done, and it showed a Meckel's diverticulum. The patient underwent a segmental resection of the terminal ileum with excellent results.

   In an anaemic patient with normal gastroscopy and a colonoscopy, it is essential to investigate further and make a diagnosis. A CTAP scan is a good starting point. Proceed to a diagnosis with a CT scan:

   - If the CT is normal and GI bleeding is thought to have occurred, other investigations such as a *Meckel's scan* or a *capsule endoscopy* may be of assistance.
   - Meckel's scan is an isotope scan that shows the presence of a Meckel's diverticulum. *It is more accurate in children than in adults.*

   The author benefitted from this earlier experience when nearly 20 years later another young man presented with identical symptoms. As double-ended endoscopy was normal a Meckel's scan was done. This confirmed the presence of a Meckel's diverticulum. A laparoscopic assisted resection of the Meckel's segment resolved the problem.

4. *Gastrointestinal bleeding in a 6-year-old child.*
   A 6-year-old child presented to the A&E department with melaena and a haemoglobin of 60 g/L. An angiogram to locate the cause of the bleeding did not yield the diagnosis. Presuming Meckel's diverticulum to be one of the most common causes of bleeding in a child, a laparotomy was done and as suspected the Meckel's diverticulum (**Figure 1**) was found and resected! Interestingly the diverticulum had a blood vessel reaching the tip of

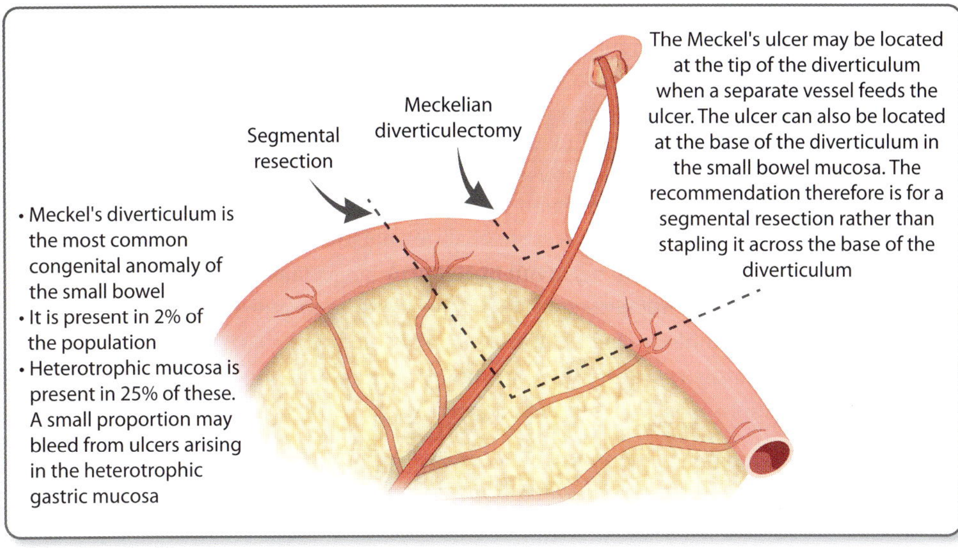

Figure 1 Meckel's diverticulum with an ulcer at the tip.

the diverticulum from which point the bleeding had occurred. A senior surgeon stated that he had seen this four times in his experience in a child and that, on every occasion, there was a separate vessel from the mesentery reaching out to the tip of the Meckel's diverticulum.

Meckel's diverticulum presentation:

- 2% of the population
- 2 feet from the ileocaecal junction
- *Two complications:* Bleeding and perforation may occur

5. *Role of NEWS/SIRS in day-to-day management. Ensure normal physiological function prior to discharge.*

   A 60-year-old patient with cardiomyopathy underwent a laparoscopic anterior resection. He was managed as per the enhanced recovery policy. He was allowed home, 5 days postoperatively. He was re-admitted on the 8th postoperative day and needed an emergency Hartmann's procedure for an anastomotic leak after which he made rapid recovery. On scrutinising the observation chart at the time of his discharge it was noted that his:

   - Heart rate (HR) was 114 beats/min
   - Temperature was 38.1°C
   - *WBC:* 12.8

Clearly the patient was in a state of systemic inflammatory response and should not have been discharged from the hospital without a clear cause for this abnormality.

- SIRS is a response to inflammation. In some it is a harbinger of sepsis
  Systemic inflammatory response syndrome
  T - Temperature: > 38°C to < 36°C
  T - Tachycardia: > 90/min

T - Tachypnoea: > 20/min
T – Total white cell count: <4 or >12 × 10^9/L
Note: Blood sugar may also be elevated in a non-diabetic. Mentation may be affected.
If two of the above four are elevated the patient is deemed to be in a state of systemic inflammatory response or SIRS.

- NEWS scoring system (Volume 1 of Snippets) is used throughout the UK to target and trigger a response. It is a score of abnormal physiology
- *If the trend over time points to abnormal physiology, then it is imperative to rule out abnormal pathology*
- Abnormal pathology leads to abnormal physiology
- If a patient is in a state of SIRS, then the patient should not be discharged without investigations to rule out abnormality

6. *Clinical examination of the abdomen and femoral hernia. Examination of the part (abdomen) always includes an examination of the groin.*
A 78-year-old lady presented to the A&E department with lower abdominal pain. She was centrally obese and suffered from memory loss. Clinical examination of the abdomen showed a soft abdomen with minimal left lower quadrant tenderness. She was discharged as all the physiological parameters were normal. Her white cell count was 11.3. She came back after 24 hours as her symptoms had not settled. This time an examination of the abdomen showed a palpable tender femoral hernia, the size of a tennis ball. CT scan confirmed a femoral hernia with small bowel obstruction. She underwent immediate surgery and resection of gangrenous small bowel.
    - No examination of the abdomen is complete without examination of all the hernial sites around the groin
    - The initial examination in the A&E department missed the obvious groin lump as it was not examined
    - Intervention early in the course of a pathological process decreases operative difficulty, morbidity and mortality

7. *Clinical examination of the abdomen and torsion testis*
Continuing from the same theme above, a 9-year-old boy was admitted with right iliac fossa pain of 3 hours duration. Clinical examination of the abdomen was normal and he was admitted for observation and assessment of progress. 4 hours later, as the pain was getting worse, he was re-examined and found to have a torsion of the right testis for which he underwent immediate surgery.
    - No examination of the abdomen is complete without examination of the external genitalia
    - Torsion of the testis can present with symptoms of pain in the right iliac fossa
    - In the absence of localising symptoms in the right iliac fossa and when appendicitis is suspected in a young male, torsion of the testis must be excluded by clinical examination

8. *Thyroglossal cyst and papillary carcinoma*
A 36-year-old lady presented with a well-defined cystic lump in the mid neck slightly to the left of the midline. The thyroid gland was not palpable. The lump moved with

the protrusion of the tongue and a clear history of the duration of the lump was not forthcoming. A clinical diagnosis of a thyroglossal cyst was made. Fine-needle aspiration cytology, however, confirmed it to be a papillary carcinoma.

- Occult papillary carcinoma of the neck may present as a cervical cyst
- Fine-needle aspiration cytology under ultrasound control is an essential part of the assessment
- This type of presentation can often lead to a delay in diagnosis of the primary thyroid carcinoma

9. *Ischaemic bowel and atrial fibrillation*
   A 63-year-old diabetic lady presented with abdominal pain. Diabetic control was reasonable. Clinical examination of the abdomen was entirely normal. There were no guarding and no areas of tenderness. The pain she stated was intermittent and severe. A diagnosis of 'non-specific abdomen,' a fashionable diagnosis, was made in the early 1980s as the only means of examination was the palpating hand. It was then noticed that her pulse was irregularly irregular. A diagnosis of atrial fibrillation was made. A laparotomy was done purely based on her severe abdominal pain. No scans of any type were available in those days. She had a dusky small bowel from just distal to the duodenojejunal (D-J) flexure to mid-ileum. The superior mesenteric pulsation was absent. A superior mesenteric artery embolectomy was very gratifying when out extruded a long length of an embolus. The bowel pinked up immediately. She was discharged home 10 days later.
   - Ischaemic bowel must be suspected when a patient with atrial fibrillation presents with abdominal pain.
   - *The other clues are:*
     - Elevated white cell count
     - Raised amylase
     - An acidosis that is refractory to correction

- Pancreatitis and ischaemic bowel can be difficult to differentiate. Persistent acidosis and imaging with CT scan will be of great assistance

10. *Appendicitis and sepsis*
    A 21-year-old lady presented after a holiday in Spain with severe abdominal pain in 1989. In Spain, the cause of her pain was attributed to eating holiday food. *No one examined her!* On arrival in the UK, the pain was worse, she called the emergency services and was assured over the phone that the pain was likely to be due to holiday food. 6 hours later her condition deteriorated. She was admitted to the hospital with a diagnosis of ectopic pregnancy. On examination of the abdomen, she had a board like rigidity and underwent an immediate laparotomy for peritonitis under antibiotic cover. The cause was a gangrenous appendix with generalised peritonitis. She recovered immediately but 6 hours later, she had full blown sepsis and multiorgan failure. This required management in the intensive care for a week before she made a gradual and prolonged recovery.
    - Gangrenous appendicitis can very rapidly proceed in certain patients to full blown sepsis with multiorgan failure
    - Current management protocols and NEWS scoring will have addressed this more quickly

- The sepsis six protocol should be initiated on suspicion of sepsis
- These patients should be managed in the HDU in the postoperative period and not in a level 1 facility such as a general ward.

The scenarios above date from the time prior to the free availability of radiological investigations. These have been discussed to bring home the point that good clinical examination can be a pointer in the right direction permitting rapid and appropriate intervention.

'*Image before intervention*' should be the rule. The need for rapid imaging and early intervention cannot be overstated.

Conclusion

Every surgical mishap carries a lesson. Some are learned early and others at great cost. It is through reflection, accountability, and adaptation that these experiences translate into safer practice and better care for future patients. If you already do not have a 'reflective diary', you should think of investing in one. In surgery, mistakes remembered and reflected upon become wisdom; those ignored are destined to recur.

Chapter 16

Multiple choice questions: Test yourself

Srinivasan Ravi

These questions are based on the author's personal experience in many aspects of general surgery.

1. A 79-year-old lady presents with a new lump in the left breast of 3 months duration. The last screening mammogram she had was 4 years ago. Your plan is:

- **a.** Clinical examination and history
- **b.** Mammogram
- **c.** Ultrasound examination
- **d.** Core biopsy if suspicious on scanning
- **e.** All of the above

2. A 28-year-old lady complains of nipple discharge which is clear. There is no relationship to periods. She is not pregnant. There is no blood in the discharge. There is no palpable lump or tenderness. There is no family history of breast cancer. The likely diagnosis is:

- **a.** Fibroadenoma
- **b.** Mastitis
- **c.** Breast cancer
- **d.** Fibrocystic disease
- **e.** Milk fistula

3. Screening mammography is done between the ages of:

- **a.** 35 and 60 years
- **b.** 49 and 75 years
- **c.** 40 and 69 years
- **d.** 50 and 80 Years
- **e.** Whenever the primary care practitioner recommends it

4. Malignant lesions of the breast are suspected on mammogram when there is:

- **a.** Microcalcification
- **b.** Oedema of the whole breast
- **c.** Linear calcification
- **d.** Well-defined rounded lesion
- **e.** Decrease in fatty tissue around the breast glands

5. A 16-year-old girl is referred with a new lump in the breast. On examination, the lump is non-tender. It is about 2 cm in diameter and is mobile and well-defined. There are no other lumps that are palpable. Clinically, this is likely to be:
   a. Fibroadenoma
   b. Fibrocystic disease
   c. Duct ectasia
   d. Mastitis
   e. Palpable lactiferous tubules

6. A 52-year-old lady has a screening mammogram. A diagnosis of cancer can be made if the mammogram shows evidence of:
   a. Microcalcification
   b. Tethering of skin
   c. Retraction of nipple
   d. Thickening of skin over a lump
   e. All of the above

7. Fine-needle cytology detects malignancy because malignant cells:
   a. Are less adherent and liable to aspiration
   b. Densely adherent and can be aspirated with suction
   c. Cancer cells can be seen with mitosis
   d. Infiltration of tissue can be confirmed
   e. The cytoplasm is large

8. In a malignant cell noted on cytology the:
   a. Nucleus is large and prominent
   b. Cytoplasm is larger than the nucleus
   c. Cell membrane is breached
   d. Mitochondria are clearly seen
   e. Nuclear cytoplasmic ratio favours the cytoplasm

9. A false positive diagnosis of breast cancer is likely to lead to anxiety and require further radiological and cytological assessment. This is more common in:
   a. Women with dense breasts
   b. Women who have had breast biopsies
   c. Women on HRT
   d. Women with a family history of breast cancer
   e. All of the above

10. False negative breast cancer on screening mammogram:
   a. Is seen in a fifth of patients who are screened
   b. Is more common in the elderly
   c. Does not have clinical significance
   d. Is reassuring
   e. Does not delay treatment

11. *P53* is referred to as the guardian of the genome because:
    - a. It is the last to mutate
    - b. It mutates early in cancers
    - c. It promotes apoptosis when there is a non-repairable mismatch
    - d. It is affected by exposure to sun light
    - e. *P53* mutation is never seen in malignancy

12. The presence of dysplasia on histology is important in the management of the patient because:
    - a. High-grade dysplasia suggests propensity to malignancy
    - b. Low-grade dysplasia shows breach of basement membrane
    - c. It is just a feature on histology of little consequence unlikely to affect the management
    - d. Shows change from columnar to squamous epithelium and further changes may follow leading to malignancy
    - e. Means the presence of mitotic cells

13. Adenocarcinoma arises from:
    - a. Cutaneous epithelium
    - b. Columnar epithelium
    - c. Mesenchymal cells
    - d. Anal canal
    - e. Proximal oesophagus

14. Lobular carcinoma of the breast:
    - a. Easily detected on mammograms
    - b. Show features of micro calcification
    - c. Difficult to detect on mammogram
    - d. Constitutes 40% of all breast cancers
    - e. Only occurs in the over 70 year olds

15. Duct carcinoma in situ (DCIS) is diagnosed histologically when:
    - a. Neoplastic cells breach the duct basement membrane
    - b. Neoplastic cells are noted localised to lobules
    - c. Neoplastic cells are contained within ducts but without breaching the basement membrane
    - d. A lump present with small lymph nodes in the axilla none measuring >0.5 cm
    - e. Primary breast lump is T1 on the TNM staging

16. Treatment options for DCIS or duct carcinoma in situ includes:
    - a. Mastectomy
    - b. Lumpectomy
    - c. Lumpectomy and radiotherapy
    - d. Lumpectomy and hormone therapy
    - e. All of the above

17. A 69-year-old man presents with a history of rectal bleeding of 4 weeks duration. On examination, he has a palpable lesion in the anal canal that infiltrates the skin. It is located between 6 and 9 o'clock positions and is non-tender. Colonoscopy was normal but this could not be biopsied because it was very low. The patient:

- **a.** Needs an examination under anaesthesia and biopsy of lesion
- **b.** Biopsy is likely to confirm squamous cell carcinoma
- **c.** MRI of the ano-rectum is needed to define the local extent
- **d.** CT scan is needed to define the systemic extent
- **e.** All of the above

18. A patient with left colonic cancer of the rectum is most likely to present with:

- **a.** Bleeding with constipation of long duration
- **b.** Bleeding with recent change in bowel habit to lose stools
- **c.** Painful defaecation
- **d.** Proctalgia fugax
- **e.** Anaemia

19. A 63-year-old Caucasian female patient is seen in the outpatient clinic with right-sided abdominal discomfort. There has been no change in his bowel habit. She has a mobile palpable mass in the iliac fossa that is non-tender. The liver is palpable and non-tender. She does not appear jaundiced. The possible diagnosis is:

- **a.** Appendicitis
- **b.** Caecal malignancy with liver secondaries
- **c.** Mucocoele of the gallbladder
- **d.** Inguinal hernia
- **e.** Rectus sheath haematoma

20. A 27-year-old man with a history of previous ulcerative colitis presents with recent rectal bleeding and loose stools. He has missed scheduled 2 yearly calls for follow-up colonoscopy. The initial presentation was at the age of 17 years with diarrhoea when pan colitis was detected. In this case:

- **a.** There is no possibility of bowel cancer at his age
- **b.** There is an increased risk of bowel cancer with increasing duration since diagnosis of total colitis
- **c.** The risk of bowel cancer is the same as for patients presenting with distal proctitis
- **d.** The history of ulcerative colitis is not linked with bowel cancer
- **e.** Reassurance and review in a few weeks should suffice

21. A 25-year-old man presents with intermittent bleeding on defaecation of 6 months duration. There is no new change in his bowel habit. The blood is sometimes noted in the pan and other times on paper but always with a bowel movement. Constipation makes the bleeding worse. The possibility here is:

- **a.** Haemorrhoids
- **b.** Fistula in ano
- **c.** Fissure in ano

d. Pilonidal sinus
e. Perianal haematoma

22. A 33-year-old lady presents with perianal discomfort. On examination, you note the presence of an external opening at about the 5 o'clock position approximately 2 cm away from the anal verge. A diagnosis of fistula in ano is made. The internal opening is most likely to be at:
a. 5 o'clock in direct continuity with the external opening
b. In the midline on the posterior aspect of the ano rectum
c. Could be located at any site on the left in the ano rectum
d. In the midline anteriorly in females
e. Can be anywhere in the ano rectum

23. A 78-year-old man presents with a rapidly progressive abdominal distension associated with constipation. His quality of life is good. Clinical examination shows a distended tympanitic abdomen with tenderness in the right lower quadrant. CT scan suggests left-sided colonic obstruction. The colonic diameter is 15 cm. There is a possibility of perforation in:
a. The transverse colon
b. In the prestenotic colon just proximal to the obstruction
c. In the caecum
d. In the poststenotic rectum
e. Limited risk of perforation

24. A 64-year-old man underwent a difficult colonoscopic caecal polypectomy in the morning. He presents to the 'Accident and Emergency (A&E)' in a moribund state with profuse rectal bleeding. The Hb at presentation is 50 and he is very confused. Pending immediate surgical intervention, this situation also calls for:
a. Massive transfusion protocol implementation
b. Routine IV fluids rapidly at 5 mL/kg
c. Another colonoscopy
d. Repeat assessment to verify the Hb
e. Immediate transfusion of O-positive blood

25. With respect to the internal anal sphincter:
a. It is the sphincter that is seen at the base of the fissure
b. Damage to this can lead to problems with incontinence in 30% of patients
c. Under anaesthesia it can be lower than the external sphincter
d. It is the whitish sphincter that is seen during haemorrhoid surgery
e. All of the above

26. Cancers occurring in the lower third of the oesophagus are:
a. Associated with *H. pylori* infections
b. Are squamous cell carcinoma
c. Are not associated with metaplasia

d. Are adenocarcinoma
e. Never linked to Barrett's oesophagus

27. A 72-year-old ex-smoker presents with new onset of dysphagia for solids. Endoscopy shows a malignant looking lesion of the oesophagus at the junction of the upper and middle third. Histological samples taken are likely to show:
    a. Adenocarcinoma
    b. Squamous cell carcinoma
    c. Barrett's mucosa with metaplastic change
    d. Oesophagitis with granulation
    e. Sarcoma

28. Distal gastric cancers have decreased over the years compared to gastro-oesophageal cancers because:
    a. The cohort of *H. pylori* infection in populations has decreased
    b. People are eating better diet
    c. Decreased consumption of smoked fish
    d. Increased consumption of red meat
    e. Regular use of lactose free milk

29. In patients with diagnosed Barrett's oesophagus, the risk of oesophageal cancer increases:
    a. With Barrett's for over 10 years
    b. Over 3 years
    c. Symptoms of reflux disease
    d. *H. pylori* infection
    e. Peptic ulceration

30. A 59-year-old man presents with an ulcer over the medial malleolus on the right. On examination, he has good peripheral pulses and prominent varicose veins in the lower limb. The skin around the ulcer is pigmented and brown.
    a. The venous ulcers are wide with sloping edges
    b. The ankle joint movements are likely to be restricted due to subcutaneous thickening
    c. The pigmentation is the result of prolonged venous hypertension leading to haemosiderin deposits
    d. Vascular ulcers are likely to look 'punched out'
    e. All of the above

31. The venous return to the heart from the peripheries is facilitated at the capillary level by:
    a. The hydrostatic pressure being greater than the osmotic pressure at the venular end
    b. The osmotic pressure being higher than the hydrostatic pressure at the arteriolar end
    c. The osmotic pressure being higher than the hydrostatic pressure at the venular end
    d. The osmotic pressure being lower than the hydrostatic pressure at the venular end
    e. Increased venous pressure leading to venous hypertension on standing

32. A 33-year-old lady presents with bleeding from a varicose ulcer. The immediate treatment involves:
   a. Diathermy of the bleeding site
   b. Ligation of the underlying vessel
   c. Cauterisation with silver nitrate
   d. Elevation and compression
   e. Tranexamic acid tablets

33. A 79-year-old lady presents with left lower abdominal pain. The diagnosis in A&E is one of diverticulitis. On examination, you note a tender swelling in the left groin. She says that this is new and has been worsening for 48 hours. The abdomen is distended. The clinical suspicion must include:
   a. Acute lymphadenitis
   b. Metastatic melanoma
   c. Diverticular abscess
   d. Obstructed femoral hernia
   e. Saphena varix

34. A 76-year-old man presents to the clinic with a large left-sided inguino scrotal swelling. On examination, there is oedema in the skin and redness. The hernia is not reducible. The possibility here is:
   a. A strangulated inguino-scrotal hernia
   b. A femoral hernia
   c. Direct inguinal hernia with bladder
   d. Epididymitis
   e. Prostatitis with epididymo-orchitis

35. A 53-year-old lady had a total abdominal hysterectomy 4 years ago for fibroids. She is referred with a new suprapubic lump of 6 months duration. Her body mass index (BMI) is 36 kg/m^2. She has a scar of a Pfannenstiel incision and a lump in the middle that is non-tender and fatty. This is most likely to be:
   a. An incisional hernia
   b. Femoral hernia
   c. Endometritis with ectopic tissue
   d. Desmoid tumour
   e. Rectus muscle haematoma

36. A 65-year-old presents with a right-groin hernia. The distinction between direct and indirect hernia is:
   a. Unimportant because the mesh repair is the same
   b. Needed to tell the patient the type of hernia
   c. Necessary as the types of mesh vary
   d. Needed as the risk of strangulation is higher with indirect hernia and surgery may be preferable
   e. Is unlikely to be of value

37. The internal ring of the inguinal canal can be surface marked for occlusion to confirm a direct hernia by its location:
   a. Half an inch above the midpoint of the inguinal ligament
   b. Half an inch above the mid-inguinal point
   c. Half an inch just below and lateral to the pubic tubercle
   d. Just above the pubic tubercle
   e. Just medial to the anterior superior iliac spine

38. The femoral hernia is bounded:
   a. Laterally by the femoral nerve outside the sheath
   b. The femoral artery medially within the femoral sheath
   c. The femoral vein laterally within the femoral sheath
   d. The lacunar ligament laterally
   e. Pectinate ligament anteriorly

39. Hiatus hernia is an internal hernia and is of two types. The sliding and the rolling – para-oesophageal hernia. The sliding hernia is a type of hernia in which:
   a. The stomach slides by the side of the gastro-oesophageal junction
   b. The gastro-oesophageal junction moves up the diaphragmatic hiatus obliterating the angle of His causing reflux
   c. The oesophagus moves distally into the abdomen accentuating the angle of His
   d. The spleen slides through the diaphragmatic defect
   e. The greater omentum is in the diaphragmatic hiatus

40. An 82-year-old lady who lives by herself presents with an acutely painful lump in the right groin. The lump was noticed by her only 2 days ago. She now complains of abdominal distension and nausea. Clinically, there is a well-defined tender lump just around the pubic tubercle. This must raise the suspicion of:
   a. An acute lymphadenitis
   b. Inflamed groin lymph node
   c. Impending strangulation in a femoral hernia
   d. Pubic osteitis
   e. A recent onset of inguinal hernia

41. A pregnant 26-year-old lady in the late second trimester presents with a swelling in the neck of a few weeks' duration. On examination, there is a diffuse lump overlying the trachea that moves with swallowing. It is non-tender and appears to indicate an enlargement of the whole of the thyroid gland. There is no tachycardia. The clinical diagnosis is likely to be:
   a. Colloid goitre
   b. Acute thyrotoxicosis
   c. Multinodular goitre
   d. Throat infection
   e. Thyroiditis

42. A 38-year-old lady presents with a thyroid nodule that is slowly increasing in size. She has previously been treated with radiotherapy to the neck when she was 19 years old for lymphoma. Clinically, there is a solitary nodule. With this history one must suspect:
    a. Papillary carcinoma
    b. Follicular carcinoma
    c. Multinodular goitre
    d. Colloid goitre
    e. Thyrotoxicosis

43. A 43-year-old lady is seen in the clinic with a neck lump that moves on swallowing. It is 4 cm in size and is in the left lobe of the thyroid. Fine needle aspiration cytology (FNAC):
    a. Sensitivity is high for follicular carcinoma
    b. Sensitivity is low for follicular carcinoma
    c. Sensitivity is low for papillary carcinoma
    d. Sensitivity for cystic lesions is higher than solid lesions
    e. Unlikely to be a useful guide

44. In a patient with a solitary nodule of the thyroid the work-up should include:
    a. Thyroid function tests
    b. Thyroid autoantibodies
    c. Ultrasound examination to distinguish between cystic and solid lesions
    d. Fine needle aspiration cytology
    e. All of the above

45. A 61-year-old lady presents with recurrent renal colic. Serum calcium is 2.8 mmol/L. This is repeated and noted to be 2.9 mmol/L. The cause for this could be:
    a. A parathyroid adenoma
    b. Carcinoma of the breast with bone metastasis
    c. Hyper parathyroidism
    d. Parathyroid hyperplasia
    e. All of the above

46. Parathormone acts to:
    a. Increase osteoclastic activity
    b. Decreases serum calcium levels
    c. Decreases absorption of calcium from the bone
    d. Decreases absorption of calcium from the gut by supressing calcitriol production
    e. Counters the action of thyroxine

47. Calcium plays an important role in the metabolism of the body because:
    a. It is involved in excitation – contraction and excitation-secretion
    b. It has a role in the coagulation process
    c. Cardiac contractility is influenced by calcium
    d. It may be a catalyst in enzymatic reactions
    e. All of the above

48. A 49-year-old lady is referred with biochemical hypercalcaemia. The parathormone levels are raised. An ultrasound examination of the neck shows a solitary nodule behind the right lobe of the thyroid. This can be:

a. Graves' disease of thyroid
b. Parathyroid adenoma
c. Parathyroid hyperplasia
d. Anaplastic thyroid carcinoma
e. Multinodular goitre

49. A 77-year-old man underwent a laparotomy for diverticular perforation and peritonitis. Five days after surgery at 6 PM the abdominal wound breaks down and there is a sero-sanguineous discharge:

a. A thorough examination of the wound to exclude dehiscence is needed
b. Change dressing to absorbent pack
c. Apply waterproof dressing
d. Reassure the patient and prescribe antibiotics
e. Advise the nurse to inform the parent team the next morning

50. At operation for a total abdominal dehiscence the skin is not approximated due to the presence of ongoing infection. This wound is likely to heal by:

a. Second intention
b. Epithelialisation
c. Contraction
d. Granulation
e. All of the above

Chapter 17

Multiple choice question: Answers

Srinivasan Ravi

1. **e.** The key principle highlighted here is 'triple assessment'. That is an examination of the breast for a suspected carcinoma is only complete with 'clinical, radiological and cytological assessment'. The radiological assessment precedes cytological assessment as the cytology is carried out under imaging where possible. Where it is not possible, and the clinician carries out the cytology, it is best to do it after radiological imaging to prevent distortion of the image.

2. **d.** Clinically the discharge is most likely to be related to fibrocystic disease; imaging is needed to confirm this. Ultrasound examination is preferable as the first step.

3. **b.** Beyond the age of 75 years screening may be carried out on request. Screening must be distinguished from follow-up mammography which is based on clinical decision and fitness of the patient. Screening mammogram before the age of 49 years is offered in some countries. In the younger people, interpretation is difficult because of the density of breast tissue and the paucity of adipose tissue.

4. **a.** By definition micro-calcification is <0.5 mm in size; any calcification larger that this is 'macrocalcification'. For microcalcification to be suspicious for malignancy, it should normally be 'pleomorphic' or of variable size and 'clustered' in an area if it is to raise the suspicion of a duct carcinoma. Cancer cells within ducts outgrow their nutrition and undergo necrosis. The necrotic tissue is calcified leading to the characteristic image seen on mammograms. These are not seen on MRI! Linear and larger calcifications can relate to benign disease and trauma as well as to blood vessels. Despite all these characteristics the findings may not be clear and may need further imaging or cytology for confirmation.

5. **a.** In young women presenting with a well-defined mobile lump fibroadenoma is a reasonable clinical diagnosis. The lump is commonly very mobile and slips away from the palpating hand so it is often referred to as the *'breast mouse'.* In general terms, under the age of 30 years it is not necessary to carry out cytological confirmation as an ultrasound examination will clearly outline the localised benign nature of the lump. These types of lumps are common in young women and seldom carry any additional risk for breast cancer. The size can fluctuate and may decrease in size after menopause when the hormonal levels regress.

6. **e.** Apart from the microcalcification discussed earlier, skin changes and nipple retraction are additional confirmatory findings that raise the probability of breast cancer. In localised inflammatory breast cancer, the skin thickening may be more obvious indicating that the disease is more advanced. A third of these women have disease that has spread to the lymph nodes.

7. **a.** Malignant cells are less adherent to each other. The original study by Papanicolaou in 1928 for exfoliative cytology was feasible in cancers of the cervix only because of the ability to extract the cells with just a spatula! A large nucleus is characteristic of abnormal cytology.

8. **a.** The nucleus cytoplasmic ratio is large indicating that in malignant cells, multiplication takes predominance over function. 'Blast' cells that are immature have larger nuclei. Multiplication is a function of the nucleus. As cells mature and become organised, the nucleus becomes smaller.

9. **e.** A *false positive* diagnosis of breast cancer causes much anxiety and can sometimes take 6 months to a year for the patient and practitioner to be reassured that there is no malignancy.

10. **a.** *A false negative* is more common than one expects and can be up to 20% of mammograms in some studies. This falsely reassures the patient that there is no malignancy and often delays treatment. This must be distinguished from *'interval cancers'* which are rapidly growing cancers that were not present in the previous mammogram.

11. **c.** *P53* activates the process of apoptosis in abnormal cells and thus preserves the genome by acting as a 'check post.' It is damaged by exposure to the sun. When there is a loss of function of *P53* due to mutation, the process of apoptosis that gets rid of cells with incomplete or improper transcription is lost and abnormal cells are permitted to multiply resulting in neoplasia. Mutation in *P53* is noted in many cancers.

12. **a.** Dysplasia is a measure of the degree of restlessness in cells. The restlessness is manifest as irregularity in cell shape and size that is confined by the basement membrane. The greater the irregularity, the higher is the grade of dysplasia and the closer is the change to malignancy which will mean a breach of the basement membrane. At times, it may be difficult to exclude malignancy and there may be a need for more than one opinion before confirming a diagnosis of high-grade dysplasia.

13. **b.** Columnar epithelium is the epithelium of the entoderm and thus lines all the derivatives of the entoderm.

14. **c.** It is *difficult to detect lobular carcinoma of the breast on mammogram* as microcalcification is not a normal feature. It may be detectable as a 'mass.' Approximately 15% of breast cancers are lobular carcinoma and the presentation may be clinical rather than screen detected.

15. **c.** Duct carcinoma in situ and lobular carcinoma in situ is the term used when abnormal cells are still located 'in situ' or 'in their original place.' Only when they move

beyond the basement membrane do they take on a sinister role of 'invasive cancer'. The distinction between in situ and invasive lesions is, therefore, paramount to the further management of these patients.

16. **e**. The treatment of a patient with 'in situ' lesions is dependent of multiple factors including the age of the patient, location, size and extent. Very often patients will need a considered decision after discussions with colleagues as happens in multidisciplinary team (MDT) meetings in the UK. Where this process is not prevalent, discussions with the oncologist, radiologist and pathologist is paramount.

17. **e**. In this type of presentation, a squamous cell carcinoma of the anal canal needs to be excluded. The anal canal lesions cannot be sampled at colonoscopy as typically the lesions are below the dentate line and by definition, therefore, very painful for a biopsy to be carried out without some form of anaesthesia. The extent of the local spread is best defined for anal and rectal cancers by way of a magnetic resonance imaging (MRI). The extent of systemic spread is assessed by a CT scan. It is worthy of note that lymphatic spread of anal lesions is to the *inguinal nodes* and not to the peritoneal nodes unless very extensive.

18. **b**. The change in bowel habit in patients with left colonic malignancies is *not* constipation but lose stools. This is possibly due to a partial hold up and bacterial overgrowth as a consequence. 'A drain that stagnates, stinks!'

19. **b**. In some parts of the world, tuberculosis (TB) of the terminal ileum must also be given consideration. In the west, where the exposure to TB is not that common even given the spread of HIV, a diagnosis of carcinoma of the right colon is a reasonable one.

20. **b**. Extent of the colitis and the duration since initial presentation determines the risk of colon cancer. The risk of bowel cancer is 5 in 100 patients with pancolitis after 10 years and about 8 in a 100 at 20 years. The risk, though, may not be considered as being too high, but possibility of colon cancer must be suspected and excluded in patients presenting with new symptoms 10 years after pancolitis.

21. **a**. Easy one this! Profuse painless bleeding is normally due to haemorrhoids. Very often as they are first-degree haemorrhoids and are, therefore, seldom seen on examination. The third-degree haemorrhoids are always seen and they must be distinguished from external haemorrhoids that are just skin tags; skin tags do not bleed. Internal haemorrhoids are the ones that bleed.

22. **b**. *Goodsall* observed that perianal fistula opening anteriorly from 9 to 3 o'clock positions drained directly in a straight line and opened internally mirroring the external position of the fistulous opening. If the external opening was in the 2 o'clock position the internal opening was also likely to be at 2 o'clock position; however, when the external opening was located in the bottom half of the clock, they mostly tended to open in the midline taking a curved route. This is the norm but as always there can be exceptions.

23. **c**. Recall the Laplace's law. If you were to blow a balloon, the first part of the balloon that distends is the middle part where it is thinnest; the pressure exerted there is

greater than at the ends of the balloon. So, it is with a colon that has a continent ileocaecal valve. The part that distends first is the part of the colon that is thinnest and has the greatest diameter... the caecum. Left-sided colonic obstructions may be complicated by a right-sided perforation making it necessary to carry out a more extensive procedure in a patient who is likely to be very ill.

24. a. The principle behind the use of a defined formula is to 'to go big early.' Critical bleeding is defined as total volume blood loss in 4 hours or 150 mL/min. This tends to happen after massive trauma and the management here is to stop the bleeding and replenish the loss. In this case, the patient was pouring out blood rectally and early organisation of massive transfusion protocol even as the patient undergoes an immediate laparotomy is likely to reduce the risk of mortality. The protocol varies in different countries but the principles are to provide blood as well as the factors needed for clotting from the outset. Tranexamic acid may also be of value. *The target is to obtain a haemoglobin of 90 g/L and a blood pressure of 90 mmHg.* Patient must also be kept warm as blood and fluids are being transfused, never letting the temperature drop below 35°C.

25. e. The whitish sphincter that is seen in the traditional operation for haemorrhoids is the internal sphincter. Keep well away from it and the recovery will be better!

26. d. The cancers in the lower third of the oesophagus are adenocarcinoma and are not related to *H. pylori* infections. It is only distal gastric cancers that are. The squamous cell carcinoma tends to occur in the ectodermal part of the oesophagus and is limited to the upper and middle third of the oesophagus.

27. b. As stated above.

28. a. As the cohort of *H. pylori* infections decreased in populations, the distal cancers of the stomach decreased in numbers. The proportion of patients presenting with gastric cancers in the presence of *H. pylori* infections is <1%. When *H. pylori* is not eradicated there is a risk of progression to peptic ulceration followed by chronic gastritis and carcinoma. Aside from this, there has also been an absolute and unexplained increase in the cancers of the cardia.

29. a. The risk of carcinoma of the cardia in patients with Barrett's oesophagus increases with metaplasia. The metaplasia that occurs in the distal oesophagus is due to acid reflux. Intestinal type of mucosa in the distal oesophagus over years leads to dysplasia that progresses from low- to high-grade over time. The risk was originally thought to be high but currently there is appreciation that while the risk is higher than the general population, it is not very high. Some argue against the need for routine surveillance of Barrett's patients.

30. e. The venous ulcers are the result of local hypoxia. Local hypoxia results from perivascular cuffing with haemosiderin that leads to pigmentation and thickening. Perivascular cuffing is the result of prolonged venous hypertension in the presence of varicose veins. Valvular incompetence leads to back pressure generated by a vertical column of blood from the heart to the heels! Perivascular cuffing with pigment affects the transfer of oxygen in the peripheries. The nature of the pathology renders these ulcers difficult to heal. Elevation is the key to decreasing the venous pressure.

31. **c**. Think about this carefully and you will understand the forces that lead to venous return. This also explains, 'why decrease in albumin causes pedal oedema'. The forces that drive the blood circulation predominantly are 'vis-a-tergo and vis-a-fronte'; push from behind (the cardiac pump) and pull from the front; the negative intrathoracic pressure sucks the blood back. This process is assisted by differences between hydrostatic and osmotic pressures at either ends of the capillaries. This is the *'Starling's law'*.

32. **d.** Immediate control of bleeding at the level of the first responder is for elevation and compression. As discussed above this decreases the pressure on the venous side of the capillary leading to control. Often this process alone controls the bleeding.

33. **d.** This patient was diagnosed as having diverticular disease because the hernial sites were not examined. No examination of the abdomen is complete without examination of the hernial sites. Sure, CT scan will make the diagnosis but only if it is requested urgently. An obstructed femoral hernia in an elderly woman can progress to strangulation rapidly leading to a high mortality (30%). Timely action and intervention saves lives.

34. **a.** You knew this, I am sure. This drives home the point that the risk of strangulation is higher in an indirect hernia than a direct hernia; higher when the hernia is irreducible and obvious when there is pain and oedema.

35. **a**. This is the most likely. I have seen desmoid tumour present like this as well as ectopic endometrial tissue. The latter is unlikely in this age group. Common things are more common; rare things are rarer.

36. **d**. It is important in elective settings to assess the possibility of strangulation and advise accordingly. An easily reducible direct hernia that pops out when standing and pops back when lying is unlikely to strangulate. This is the common type in the elderly; presence of a hernia is not an indication to proceed to surgery. It is, as always, the symptoms and signs that dictate need for intervention.

37. **a**. As above it is good to differentiate between the direct and the indirect hernia in the elective setting. Operation is the same but the advice will vary.

38. **c**. The femoral vein is lateral to the femoral hernia. When we were trainees, we used to be told to 'protect the vein with the finger as you repair the defect and going through the finger with the needle is better than going through the vein'! This is not to be done. The point is made that the vein is in close approximation laterally and needs to be protected both from needle and narrowing; too tight a repair constricts the vein leading to obvious consequences.

39. **b**. A sliding hernia is classically defined as a hernia in which the viscera forms part of the sac. This is true of sliding inguinal hernia too, especially on the left when sigmoid colon is likely to be part of the wall of the sac. In case of the sliding oesophageal

hernia the stomach moves into the hernia that protrudes into the thoracic cavity. The para-oesophageal hernia protrudes through a diaphragmatic defect, through tears or through the defects of *Bochdalek* (B for back – posterior diaphragmatic defect) and *Morgagni* (anterior).

40. c. It is easy to overlook a femoral hernia. It cannot be overstated that no examination of the abdomen is complete without examination of the hernial sites and in males, the scrotum.

41. a. Colloid or pregnancy goitres occur more commonly in areas of iodine deficiency. In pregnancy, there is a greater renal elimination of iodine altering the inorganic iodine levels without changing the free thyroxine levels. These do not need surgery as they are physiological goitres. This type of goitre was originally noted in the iodine-deficient struma river valley in Bulgaria.

42. a. The relationship with radiation especially in the younger age and papillary carcinoma of the thyroid is well-established. After chernobyl nuclear disaster, the rate of thyroid cancers increased in the surrounding community. Iglesias ML, Schmidt A, Ghuzlan AA, et al. Radiation exposure and thyroid cancer: a review. Arch Endocrinol Metab 2017; 61:180–187.

43. b. The sensitivity is low for a follicular carcinoma as compared to a papillary carcinoma. Morphology alone is not sufficient to make a diagnosis of follicular cancer of the thyroid. *The diagnosis of follicular cancer is made on the basis of vascular and capsular invasion.* Neither of this is possible on cytology nor it requires a histology. Cystic lesions of the thyroid have a low sensitivity for diagnosis of cancer than solid lesions as they may only aspirate necrotic debris, blood or fluid.

44. e. Do not forget the thyroid autoantibodies as Hashimoto's thyroiditis may be picked up on this test alone. Fine-needle aspiration cytology (FNAC) is also very good at making the diagnosis of inflammatory goitres.

45. e. All these are causes of hypercalcaemia. In metastatic bone disease, the calcium levels can be elevated.

46. a. Parathormone works to increase the calcium levels by also acting on the kidney to retain the calcium as well as increasing absorption from bowel by stimulating calcitriol.

47. e. Calcium is a major player in the metabolic world!

48. b. Parathyroid adenoma is mostly single while hyperplasia affects all the parathyroid glands.

49. a. The early sign of dehiscence of the abdominal wound is a light sero-sanguinous discharge. It is important as this stage to rule out infection as well as possible dehiscence. If there is dehiscence and the patient is suitable for return to theatre for re-exploration, this must be done expeditiously. In some situations, the bowel may be totally adherent to the abdominal wall making immediate intra-abdominal exploration technically difficult. A CT scan may assist in ensuring that there is no deep cavity infection. In patients who have had a resection anastomosis, exclusion of anastomotic leak is needed.

50. **e**. All these processes are important. The wound contraction acts to decrease the circumference, thus, reducing the area needing to be bridged by the epithelium over sprouting granulation that fills the pit! Sprout, pull and bridge the reducing gap. Marvellous process!.

Chapter 18

Reflections on progress in surgery – surgery then and now

Srinivasan Ravi

Introduction

The delivery of surgical care has undergone a monumental change in the last half century. The progress in surgery can be divided into two eras of before and after technological impact:

1. The era of changes in surgical techniques
2. The era of changes in surgical technology

Until the advent of new technology all the changes in surgery were limited to discussions and implementation of variations in techniques. Progress meant doing a selective or highly selective vagotomy instead of truncal vagotomy; using nylon instead of silk or thread; vicryl instead of catgut. The power of the clinical assessment and the examining hand was supreme. There was little if any other form of assistance in making the diagnosis other than routine blood counts and chest X-ray initially. Subsequent progress ushered in barium examinations of the bowel. Gastro-oesophagoscopy was limited to examining the oesophagus and proximal stomach with a poorly lighted rigid tube and under general anaesthesia. I recall carrying out these examinations with tubes similar to a rigid sigmoidoscope. Invariably the bulb lighting the tube would fuse at the exact moment of taking a biopsy! How things have changed!

Then came major advances in imaging, in the late 1970s starting with ultrasonography, followed rapidly in the early 1980s by computerised tomography and magnetic resonance imaging. Concurrently, there was the invention of the video camera, fibre optics, rod-lens system and colour television. This was soon followed by miniaturisation. The fibre optics brought in gastroscopes and colonoscopes; the light source could be placed away and transmitted with fibre optic tubes that were flexible. Miniature video cameras connected to a screen meant better quality of imaging, easier training, and greater transparency.

In the absence of assistance from technology patients were subjected to operations based on subjective and clinical assessment alone. I recall ward rounds in mid-1970s where the consultant would examine the patient who presented with upper abdominal pain. If there was a deep tender spot in the epigastrium on palpation, the patient would be quizzed on the duration of symptoms. If the duration exceeded, 3 years, the patient would be listed for a gastrojejunostomy and vagotomy (GJ and V). If it was present for less than a year, the patient would be sent home on antacids and dietary advice. If it was in between 1 and 3 years, depending on availability, a barium meal examination of the stomach would be requested. The ulcers, if present, would be seen clearly in the duodenum as a pit or puckering with radiation away from it. Gastric ulcers, likewise.

There would be lots of discussions on the images. The gastric cancers would be seen as space occupying lesions. Sometimes there would be 'pyloric stenosis.' With duodenal ulcers, this is used to be a common presentation with a clearly visible gastric peristalsis which moved in the epigastrium from left to right. The stenosis would always be in the first part of the duodenum unlike the gastric cancers which would be more proximal.

The fitness for surgery depended on the surgeon's assessment. This always considered the age of the patient, the duration that the patient could hold the breath and the ability to walk up a flight of stairs.

The operations proceeded at a very rapid pace as the anaesthetic support was quite different. The muscle relaxants were variable. The exposure was limited consequently. After a truncal vagotomy, the gastrojejunostomy in two layers would be carried out in the retrocolic plane and in an isoperistaltic direction with a short loop of the duodenum. The material was always either catgut or chromic catgut. The antibiotic cover was restricted to penicillin or strepto-penicillin. The laparotomy wound would be closed with thread or silk in layers. The skin would be approximated with either vertical mattress or simple sutures. Occasionally, continuous silk or nylon would be used with a straight needle that would be threaded by the theatre nurse.

Dressings were with gauze or Gamjee pads that were made of a sandwich of cotton between two layers of gauze. *The wards had a 'dresser'* employed by the hospital who would ensure that the instruments used for the dressings would be kept sterile. Some were kept soaked in a solution of 'Dettol.'

In the absence of technological progress many patients underwent needless laparotomies. For instance, the indication for cholecystectomy was again purely based on clinical assessment. If the patient had a palpable gallbladder in the presence of jaundice, then it was deemed to be secondary to pancreatic malignancy. So, those patients would be subject to a triple bypass operation which consisted of choledochojejunostomy, which drained the bile duct and addressed the jaundice, jejuno-jejunostomy that ensured, distal passage of bile and a gastrojejunostomy that diverted gastric contents away from the duodenum lest it gets obstructed by the pancreatic malignanacy. Many of these patients survived less than 6 months. If the patient was suspected of having an acute cholecystitis and Murphy's sign positive the patient was treated with antibiotics until the acute symptoms resolved. They would then be discharged and brought back for an interval cholecystectomy about 3 months later. Patients with biliary colic seldom had operative intervention. If the suspicion was strong that the patient had gallstones a laparotomy would be done through a right paramedian incision. The gallbladder would be palpated for stones and if stones were not detected an appendicectomy would be carried out as a matter of routine in some surgeons' practice. For emergency, complications such as peritonitis a mid-midline laparotomy would be carried out through what was referred to as the *incision of indecision.* This could then be extended superiorly or inferiorly depending upon the findings. This meant that many patients with perforated viscous secondary to malignancies add needless laparotomies.

Reshaping of surgery with revolution in technology. Advent of technological assistance

Many factors have made a big impact on the nature of elective and emergency surgery. Here, I have discussed but a few.

1. *The advent and popularisation of electrosurgery:* Electrosurgery to cut, coagulate, desiccate, and fulgurate. Although the first commercial use is credited to *William Bowie* who worked at Harvard University between 1914 and 1927 it became popular

only towards the latter half of the last century. It is stated that *Harvey Cushing* was one of the first persons to use the diathermy machine for extracting highly vascular tumours. Currently, almost all major operations are carried out with the assistance of Electro country. This has led to less ligatures and bleeding during surgery and has enabled surgery to be carried out in clean bloodless planes where possible ultimately providing much better results for the patient.

2. *Progress in imaging:* This has been remarkable enabling diagnosis prior to intervention. Radiological progress from simple tomography to computerised tomography in the form of CT scans that can be done very quickly and with great accuracy has been of assistance not only in *making diagnoses* but also in enabling *selection of patients* suitable for surgery when required. Along with this the impact of ultrasound examinations on diagnosis not only of gallstones but also on the presence or absence of collections within the peritoneal cavity has changed the face of surgical assessment. *Magnetic resonance imaging* in the late 1980s has contributed very significantly to the diagnostic potential of imaging. Radioisotopes have enabled positron emission tomography (PET)-CT scans to be undertaken and these have added to our armamentarium in the treatment of many cancers.
3. *The recognition of H. pylori as the cause of duodenal ulcer*: This single factor alone has contributed to patient welfare by decimating surgery for peptic ulcer disease. Once the causative agent was identified in 1984 by *Marshall;* it was only a question of time before antibiotics and treatment of peptic ulcer without the need surgery was put in place. This was also assisted by the prior discovery of H_2*-blockers* in the form of *cimetidine* which reduced the gastric acid output. This reduced the need for surgical intervention in many patients. Very soon it was followed by *proton-pump inhibitors* which along with antibiotics significantly reduced the need for surgical intervention. The previous generation of surgeons was trained to do vagotomy and gastrojejunostomy or pyloroplasty. In a single stroke, these operations ceased to exist as routine procedures and became the preserve of a new generation of cosmetic bariatric surgeons. The latter is now being threatened by GLP-1 RA drugs that reduce BMI and may obviate the need for such interventional surgery.
4. *The invention of the video camera* and its miniaturisation assisted by changes in *fibre optics* (glass is a better conductor of light than air) with the use of the renowned *Harold Hopkins* invention of the *rod-lens system* ushered in *minimally invasive surgery.* His many inventions are in daily use throughout the world. These include *zoom lenses, coherent fibre-optics* and more recently the *rod-lens endoscopes* which 'opened the door' to modern key-hole surgery.

   The impact of operating through tiny incisions using small tubes and delicate instruments on postoperative pain and recovery is immense. With the absence of rummaging in the abdominal cavity that was routine following any laparotomy and with minimal access, postoperative pain control became much easier. The patients were able to move very soon after major surgery and, therefore, length of stay in the hospitals decreased significantly. This shifted routine surgery from inpatient operations to day patient procedures thereby by decreasing the number of beds needed to care for patients.
5. *Progress in anaesthetic monitoring* and delivery of anaesthesia have also made a phenomenal impact on surgery. Added to this is the current practice of assessing fitness of patients for surgery with the *cardiopulmonary exercise test.* This has

shifted the focus on physiological changes that could be put into place by way of *prehabilitation* prior to surgery.

6. *The impact of NEWS* – 'National Early Warning Scoring' system cannot be understated. It allows the patient's progress to be monitored in the wards and enables early recognition of possible complications by the principle of *'track and trigger.'* When physiological variables stray away from the norm these are recognised, and early actions enabled.
7. *Robotic surgery:* Although it is referred to as 'robotic surgery', it is truly a robotic device-assisted surgery. It is a type of minimally invasive surgery in which the surgeon uses the device to perform the surgery. The benefits of robotic surgery over laparoscopic surgery are that it is more precise. *Visibility* is better for the surgeon. In all types of minimally invasive surgery, there is likely to be less bleeding. For certain operations, the access and the view provided by robotic-assisted surgery is greater than laparoscopic surgery. It has clear benefits for certain types of operations especially ones such as radical prostatectomy and low anterior resection. There is not much of a difference between robotic and laparoscopic surgery in terms of length of stay, wound infections and complications.

In a recent study published in the Lancet in 2024, the authors conclude '*In a single centre trial of adults undergoing minimally invasive hepatectomy for liver malignancies, we observed no statistically significant differences in the functioning scale within 90 days after surgery between robotic hepatectomy (RH) and laparoscopic hepatectomy (LH). Postoperative morbidity was comparable in both groups with regard to the "Comprehensive complications index. While the LH group required more frequent postoperative interventions, we found no significant differences in posthepatectomy-specific outcomes. Moreover, there were no observed changes in postoperative recovery or other QoL outcomes between the study groups.*'

The conclusion (**Table 1**) is that robotic hepatectomy is as good as laparoscopic hepatectomy. For prostatic resections, however, it remains far superior. The visibility of the plane of dissection and the pelvic nerves is excellent with robotic surgery. Recovery time is shorter and the urethral anastomosis is very sound.

There are clearly benefits for certain types of operations over others with robotic surgery. It seems rational, therefore, to make it available for specific operations in specific

Table 1 The conclusion for the robotic surgery.

Parameter	Robotic	Laparoscopic
Visibility	Excellent	Good
Precision	Very high	High
Duration of surgery	+++	++
Set-up time	Longer	Less
Undocking time	Longer. May impede resuscitation	Less
Length of stay	No difference	
Morbidity	Similar	
Costs	More expensive	Less expensive

sites lest the costs of healthcare become exponentially higher with universal use of robotic surgery.

The operative duration is also much higher as there is added time in setting up the robotic procedure.

Access to the patient in times of emergency is also likely to be impeded with robotic surgery.

In one study, the length of stay after robotic surgery for all types of operation was 3.0 compared to 3.3 for laparoscopic surgery.

In the future, with decreasing costs and increasing training, the usage of robotics in surgery may become more widespread. Currently, the advantages for universal implementation of robotic surgery have benefits in the margin when applied to all operations in general instead of selective procedures.

In conclusion, the integration of advanced technologies into surgical practice has profoundly reshaped the discipline, establishing new paradigms of precision, efficiency, and patient safety. Innovations such as laparoscopic surgery, endoscopy, robotic-assisted systems, enhanced imaging modalities, and more recently artificial intelligence have not only expanded the scope of surgical interventions but also minimised invasiveness, reduced complication rates, and accelerated recovery times. Beyond the operating theatre, technology has streamlined preoperative planning and postoperative monitoring, thereby reinforcing continuity of care and improving long-term outcomes. The transformative impact of technology on surgery, with paradigm shifts in the immunological managements of cancers, with AI mediated diagnostics, the future direction and progress in healthcare will be changed forever.

Bibliography

Alkhayyat M, Kumar P, Sanaka KO, et al. Chemoprevention in Barrett's esophagus and esophageal adenocarcinoma. Therap Adv Gastroenterol 2021; 14:17562848211033730.

Ambrus JL, Ambrus CM, Mink IB, Pickren JW. Causes of death in cancer patients. J Med 1975; 6:61–64.

American Cancer Society. (2024a). Esophagus cancer. [online] Available from https://www.cancer.org/cancer/types/esophagus-cancer.html [Last accessed 4 February 2026].

American Cancer Society. (2024b). Stomach cancer. [online] Available from https://www.cancer.org/cancer/types/stomach-cancer.html [Last accessed 4 February 2026].

American Joint Committee on Cancer. Esophagus and esophagogastric junction. In: Amin MB, Greene FL, Edge SB, et al. (eds), AJCC cancer staging manual, 8th edn. New York: Springer, 2016a:185–202.

American Joint Committee on Cancer. Stomach. In: Amin MB, Greene FL, Edge SB, et al. (eds), AJCC cancer staging manual, 8th edn. New York: Springer, 2016b:203–220.

Andrade C. Misunderstandings, explanations, challenges, and alternatives. Indian J Psychol Med 2019; 41:210–215.

Arnold M, Abnet CC, Neale RE, et al. Global burden of five major gastrointestinal cancers. Gastroenterology 2020; 159:335–349.e15.

Bailey JA, Weller J, Chapman CJ, et al. Faecal immunochemical testing and blood tests for prioritization of urgent colorectal cancer referrals in symptomatic patients. BJS Open 2021; 5:zraa056.

Bak MTJ, Ruiterkamp MFE, van Ruler O, et al. Prehabilitation prior to intestinal resection in Crohn's disease patients: an opinion review. World J Gastroenterol 2022; 28:2403–2416.

Barsouk A, Rawla P, Barsouk A, et al. Epidemiology of cancers of the small intestine: trends, risk factors, and prevention. Med Sci 2019; 7:46.

Berlana D. Parenteral nutrition overview. Nutrients 2022; 14:4480.

Best practice The faculty of Intensive care medicine, UK 2024.

Beydoun AS, Stabenau KA, Altman KW, Johnston N. Cancer risk in Barrett's esophagus: a clinical review. Int J Mol Sci 2023; 24:6018.

Birgin E, Heibel M, Hetjens S, et al. Robotic versus laparoscopic hepatectomy for liver malignancies (ROC'N'ROLL): a single-centre, randomised, controlled, single-blinded clinical trial. Lancet Reg Health Eur 202; 43:100972.

Blackburn WD Jr. Validity of acute phase proteins as markers of disease activity. J Rheumatol Suppl 1994; 42:9–13.

Bohnen JD, Mavros MN, Ramly EP, et al. Intraoperative adverse events in abdominal surgery: what happens in the operating room does not stay in the operating room. Ann Surg 2017; 265:1119–1125.

Boland CR, Lynch HT. The history of Lynch syndrome. Fam Cancer 2013; 12:145–157.

Boullata JI, Carrera AL, Harvey L, et al. ASPEN safe practices for enteral nutrition therapy [Formula: see text]. JPEN J Parenter Enteral Nutr. 2017; 41:15–103.

Bourgault AM, Xie R, Talbert S, et al. Association of enteral feeding with microaspiration in critically ill adults. Appl Nurs Res 2022; 67:151611.

Burden S, Todd C, Hill J, et al. Pre-operative nutrition support in patients undergoing gastrointestinal surgery. Cochrane Database Syst Rev 2012; 11:CD008879.

Cancer Medicine: "Open access review. Has tumour doubling time in breast cancer changed over the past 80 years? A systematic review.

Cancer Research UK. (2018). Oesophageal cancer risk. [online] Available from https://www.cancerresearchuk.org [Last accessed 4 February 2026].

Cancer Research UK. (2023). Small intestine cancer incidence statistics. [online] Available from https://www.cancerresearchuk.org [Last accessed 4 February 2026].

Centers for Disease Control and Prevention (CDC) (n.d.). Breast cancer. [online] Available from https://www.cdc.gov [Last accessed 4 February 2026].

Chan AOO, Wong BC. (2024). Gastric cancer screening. UpToDate. [online] Available from https://www.uptodate.com [Last accessed 4 February 2026].

Chia SK, Wolff AC. With maturity comes confidence: EBCTCG tamoxifen update. Lancet. 2011; 378:747–749.

Clancy S. DNA damage and repair: mechanisms for maintaining DNA integrity. Nat Educ 2008; 1:103.

Cloyd JM, George E, Visser BC. Duodenal adenocarcinoma: advances in diagnosis and surgical management. World J Gastrointest Surg 2016; 8:212.

Cross AJ, Leitzmann MF, Subar AF, et al. A prospective study of meat and fat intake in relation to small intestinal cancer. Cancer Res 2008; 68:9274–9279.

Day DW, Morson BC. The adenoma–carcinoma sequence. Major Prob Pathol 1978; 10:58–71.

Delaney CP, Fazio VW, Senagore AJ, et al. Fast-track postoperative management protocol for patients with high co-morbidity undergoing complex abdominal and pelvic colorectal surgery. Br J Surg 2001; 88:1533–1538.

Delaunoit T, Neczyporenko F, Limburg PJ, et al. Pathogenesis and risk factors of small bowel adenocarcinoma: a colorectal cancer sibling? Am J Gastroenterol 2005; 100:703–710.

Early Breast Cancer Trialists' Collaborative Group. Aromatase inhibitors versus tamoxifen in early breast cancer. Lancet 2015; 386:1341–1352.

Early Breast Cancer Trialists' Collaborative Group. Effect of radiotherapy after breast-conserving surgery on recurrence and mortality. Lancet 2011; 378:1707–1716.

Erlandsson J, Holm T, Pettersson D, et al. Optimal fractionation of preoperative radiotherapy and timing to surgery for rectal cancer (Stockholm III): a multicentre, randomised, non-blinded, phase 3, non-inferiority trial. Lancet Oncol. 2017; 18:336–346.

Fisher B, Anderson S, Bryant J, et al. Twenty-year follow-up of a randomized trial comparing total mastectomy, lumpectomy, and lumpectomy plus irradiation for the treatment of invasive breast cancer. N Engl J Med 2002; 347:1233–1241.

Fleming MA 2nd, Ehsan L, Moore SR, Levin DE. The Enteric Nervous System and Its Emerging Role as a Therapeutic Target. Gastroenterol Res Pract. 2020; 2020:8024171.

Gauvreau K, Pagano M. Why 5%? Nutrition 1994; 10:93–94.

Gough D, Thomas J, Oliver S. Clarifying differences between reviews within evidence ecosystems. Syst Rev 2019; 8:170.

Gralow JR, Barlow WE, Paterson AHG, et al. Phase III randomized trial of bisphosphonates as adjuvant therapy in breast cancer (S0307). J Natl Cancer Inst 2020; 112:698–707.

Habr-Gama A, Perez RO, Nadalin W, et al. Operative versus nonoperative treatment for stage 0 distal rectal cancer following chemoradiation therapy: long-term results. Ann Surg 2004; 240:711–718.

Hardy PA, Zacharias H. Reappraisal of the Hansemann–Boveri hypothesis on the origin of tumours. Cell Biol Int 2005; 29:983–992.

Haybittle JL, Blamey RW, Elston CW, Johnson J, Doyle PJ, Campbell FC, et al. A prognostic index in primary breast cancer. Br J Cancer 1982; 45:361–366.

Hirbe AC, Gutmann DH. Neurofibromatosis type 1: a multidisciplinary approach to care. Lancet Neurol 2014; 13:834–843.

https://doi.org/10.1097%2F00000658-199908000-00006.

Huckleberry Y. Nutritional support and the surgical patient. Am J Health Syst Pharm 2004; 61:671–682.

Hussain N, Bookwala A, Sancheti P, Bhandari M. The 3-min appraisal of a meta-analysis. Indian J Orthopaed 2011; 45:4–5.

International Agency for Research on Cancer (2022). Global cancer observatory. [online] Available from https://gco.iarc.fr [Last accessed t February 2026].

Joensson A, Bhandari M. (n.d.) Clinical research for surgeons. Stuttgart: Thieme, 2009.

Kaerlev L, Teglbjaerg PS, Sabroe S, et al. Occupational risk factors for small bowel carcinoid tumour: a European population-based case–control study. J Occup Environ Med 2002; 44:516–522.

Khan K, Peckitt C, Sclafani F, et al. Prognostic factors and treatment outcomes in patients with small bowel adenocarcinoma (SBA): the Royal Marsden Hospital (RMH) experience. BMC Cancer 2015; 15:112.

Kim JJ. Upper gastrointestinal cancer and reflux disease. J Gast Cancer 2013; 13:79–85.

Krag DN, Anderson SJ, Julian TB, Brown AM, Harlow SP, Ashikaga T, et al. Technical outcomes of sentinel-lymph-node resection and conventional axillary-lymph-node dissection in patients with clinically node-negative breast cancer: results from the NSABP B-32 randomised phase III trial. Lancet Oncol 2007; 8:881–888.

Krag DN, Anderson SJ, Julian TB, et al. Sentinel-lymph-node resection compared with conventional axillary-lymph-node dissection in clinically node-negative patients with breast cancer: overall survival findings from the NSABP B-32 randomised phase 3 trial. Lancet Oncol 2010; 11:927–933.

Larke NL, Thomas SL, dos Santos Silva I, et al. Male circumcision and penile cancer: a systematic review and meta-analysis. Cancer Causes Control 2011; 22:1097–1110.

Ljungqvist O, Scott M, Fearon KC. Enhanced recovery after surgery: a review. JAMA Surg 2017; 152:292–298.

Locher C, Batumona B, Afchain P, et al. Small bowel adenocarcinoma: French intergroup clinical practice guidelines for diagnosis, treatments and follow-up (SNFGE, FFCD, GERCOR, UNICANCER, SFCD, SFED, SFRO). Dig Liver Dis 2018; 50:15–19.

Melzack R, Wall PD. Pain mechanisms: a new theory. Science 1965; 150:971–979.

Monahan KJ, Bradshaw N, Dolwani S, et al. Guidelines for the management of hereditary colorectal cancer from the British Society of Gastroenterology (BSG)/Association of Coloproctology of Great Britain and Ireland (ACPGBI)/United Kingdom Cancer Genetics Group (UKCGG). Gut 2020; 69:411–444.

Mordecai Schwartz D. Cancer. Wiley Online Library. 1961.

Mukherjee S. The emperor of all maladies: a biography of cancer. New York: Scribner, 2010.

National Academies Press. Ensuring the integrity of the research process: Volume I. Washington (DC): National Academies Press, 1992.

National Institute for Health and Care Excellence (NICE). (2021). Gastrointestinal tract (upper) cancers – recognition and referral. [online] Available from https://cks.nice.org.uk [Last accessed 4 February 2026].

Nicholson BD, Shinkins B, Pathiraja I, et al. Blood CEA levels for detecting recurrent colorectal cancer. Cochrane Database Syst Rev 2015; 2015:CD011134.

Nigro ND. An evaluation of combined therapy for squamous cell cancer of the anal canal. Dis Colon Rectum 1984; 27:763–766.

Oka P, Sidhu R. Small bowel lymphoma. Curr Opin Gastroenterol 2022; 38:270–278.

Oxford Centre for Evidence-Based Medicine (n.d.) Numbers needed to treat. [online] Available from https://www.cebm.ox.ac.uk [Last accessed: 4 February 2026].

Palma GD De.Management strategies of Barrett's esophagus. World J Gastroenterol 2012; 18:6216–6225.

Pandya K, Overman MJ, Gulhati P. Molecular landscape of small bowel adenocarcinoma. Cancers 2022; 14:1287.

Pastino A, Lakra A. Patient-Controlled Analgesia. 2023. In: StatPearls [Internet]. Treasure Island (FL): StatPearls Publishing; 2025. PMID: 31869074.

Petras RE, Frankel WL. Large Intestine (Colon). Modern Surgical Pathology. 2009:755–836.

Schatzkin A, Park Y, Leitzmann MF, et al. Prospective study of dietary fibre, whole grain foods, and small intestinal cancer. Gastroenterology 2008; 135:1163–1167.

Schottenfeld D, Beebe-Dimmer JL, Vigneau FD. The epidemiology and pathogenesis of neoplasia in the small intestine. Ann Epidemiol 2009; 19:58–69.

Shaheen NJ. Risk of cancer in patients with Barrett esophagus. Gastroenterol Hepatol 2019; 15:688–690.

Sharma P, Dent J, Armstrong D, et al. The development and validation of an endoscopic grading system for Barrett's esophagus: the Prague C & M criteria. Gastroenterology 2006; 131:1392–1399.

Shay JW, Wright WE. Hayflick, his limit, and cellular ageing. Nature Rev Molecul Cell Biol 2000;1:72–76.

Sinn HP, Kreipe H. A brief overview of the WHO classification of breast tumors. Breast Care 2013; 8:149–154.

Sriram BM. Oesophagus. In: Sriram BM (ed.), SRB's manual of surgery, 6th edn. New Delhi: Jaypee Brothers Medical Publishers (P) Ltd., 2019a:776–803.

Sriram BM. Stomach. In: Sriram BM (ed.), SRB's manual of surgery, 6th edn. New Delhi: Jaypee Brothers Medical Publishers (P) Ltd., 2019b:804–851.

Strosberg JR, Halfdanarson TR, Bellizzi AM, et al. The North American Neuroendocrine Tumor Society consensus guidelines for surveillance and medical management of midgut neuroendocrine tumors. Pancreas 2017; 46:707–714.

Stryker SJ, Wolff BG, Culp CE, et al. Natural history of untreated colonic polyps. Gastroenterology 1987; 93:1009.

Sung H, Ferlay J, Siegel RL, et al. Global cancer statistics 2020: GLOBOCAN estimates of incidence and mortality worldwide. CA: A Cancer J Clin 2021; 71:209–249.

Swerdloff RS, Ng JCM. Gynecomastia: etiology, diagnosis, and treatment. In: Feingold KR et al. (eds), Endotext. South Dartmouth, MA: MDText.com, 2023.

Tanaka A, Yatabe T, Suhara T, et al. The optimal glycemic target in critically ill patients: an updated network meta-analysis. J Intensive Care. 2024; 12:14.

Timbres J, Kohut K, Caneppele M, et al. DCIS and LCIS: are the risk factors for developing in situ breast cancer different? Cancers 2023; 15:4397.

Todd JH, Dowle C, Williams MR, et al. Confirmation of a prognostic index in primary breast cancer. Br J Cancer 1987; 56:489–492.

Turrentine FE, Wang H, Simpson VB, et al. Surgical risk factors, morbidity, and mortality in elderly patients. J Am Coll Surg 2006; 203:865–877.

Vinik AI, Chaya C. Clinical presentation and diagnosis of neuroendocrine tumors. Hematol Oncol Clin North Am 2016; 30:21–48.

Vinik AI, Silva MP, Woltering EA, et al. Biochemical testing for neuroendocrine tumors. Pancreas 2009; 38:876–889.

Weusten BLAM, Bisschops R, Dinis-Ribeiro M, et al. Diagnosis and management of Barrett esophagus: ESGE guideline. Endoscopy 2023; 55:1124–1146.

Wind J, Polle SW, Fung Kon Jin PH, et al. Systematic review of enhanced recovery programmes in colonic surgery. Br J Surg 2006; 93:800–809.

Wolters R, Wöckel A, Janni W, et al. Comparing the outcome between multicentric and multifocal breast cancer: what is the impact on survival, and is there a role for guideline-adherent adjuvant therapy? A retrospective multicenter cohort study of 8,935 patients. Breast Cancer Res Treat 2013; 142:579–590.

Zhao Z, Feng Q, Yin Z, et al. Red and processed meat consumption and colorectal cancer risk: a systematic review and meta-analysis. Oncotarget 2017; 8:83306–83314.

Zhong L, Liu J, Liu S, et al. Correlation between pancreatic cancer and metabolic syndrome: a systematic review and meta-analysis. Front Endocrinol (Lausanne). 2023; 14:1116582.

Zugasti I, Espinosa-Aroca L, Fidyt K, et al. CAR-T cell therapy for cancer: current challenges and future directions. Signal Transduct Target Ther 2025; 10:210.

Index

Note: Page numbers in **bold** or *italic* refer to tables or figures respectively.

A

Abdomen 184
Abdomino-perineal resection 38, 113, 114
Absolute risk reduction 15
Acanthosis nigricans 67
Acquired mutation 23
Acral lentiginous melanoma 163
Acute phase proteins 154
  response 154
Additional breast imaging modalities 46
Additional therapy 55
Adenocarcinoma 62, 84, 86
Adenomas 105, 139
Adenomatous polyposis coli gene 102
Adenosine triphosphate 145
Adjuvant therapy 55
Adrenaline 176
Adrenocorticotropic hormone 156
Advanced disease 66, 74
Aflatoxin 89
Ageing and immuno-suppression 164
Alcohol
  consumption 63
  intake, excessive 89
Alkylating agents 32
Allograft 166
Alpha-fetoprotein 68, 89, 90
Amelanotic melanoma 163
Amino acids 145
Ampulla of Vater 86
Amsterdam criteria 100
  modified 100
Anabolic phase 153
Anabolic response 154
Anaemia 66, 182
Anaesthetic monitoring 206
Anal canal 120
  cancer 119
Analgesia, patient-controlled 175
Anaplastic carcinoma 135
Anaplastic thyroid cancer *136*
Anastomotic leak 118
Anterior resection 111, 113, 114
Antimetabolites 32
Antitumour antibodies 32
Anxiety 78
APC gene 63, 101-103
APC suppressor gene 102
Apnoea 179
Apoptosis 21
Appendicitis 185
Aromatase inhibitors 58
Ascending colon cancers 115
Aspiration 148, 149
  pneumonia 148
Aspirin 175
Atelectasis 148
Atrial fibrillation 185
Axilla, ultrasound evaluation of 46

B

Balanitis 167
Balanoposthitis 167
Barrat's oesophagus 63-65, 73
  pathophysiology of 64
  risk factors for 64
Basal cell carcinoma 163
Basal metabolic rate 142, 143
Bell curve 4
Biliary obstruction 66
Binomial distribution 3
Bisphosphonates, adjuvant 58
Blood
  supply *61*
  vessels, short 168
Body mass index 143
  ranges 143
Bone metastases 78
Bowel cancer screening 106
Brachial artery 180

Bradykinin 174
Brain, development of 128
BRCA mutations 63
Breast
- abscess 41, 42
- basic anatomy of *39*
- carcinoma of 43
- differences between 46
- disease 39
- lobule of *40*
- mouse 41
- reconstruction 54
- resecting surgery 54
- structure of *40*

Breast cancer 29, 41, 48
- cells 49
- genes 50
- hormone receptors, relevance of 58
- identification of *49*
- pathology 43
- presentation of 45
- risk factors for 44
- risk reduction for 44
- screening for 52
  - origins of 52
- survival 58
  - after 51, *52*
- TNM for 34, 46, *47*
- treatment of 54
  - options for 54
- triple negative 50
- types of 44

Breast conserving surgery 54, 58
- radiotherapy after 58

Breast lumps 39, *45*
- investigations for 45

Breslow's staging *162*
Bromage scale 177
Bupivacaine hydrochloride 176
Burn 164
- extent of 164
- types of 164

C

CA 19-9 68, 94
Cachexia 37
Café-au-lait spots 160
Calcidiol 138
Calcitonin 137, *139*
Calcitriol 138
Calcium *138*
- homeostasis 141
- metabolism 137

Cancer 19
- causation of 24
- cells 22, 28
- classical theory of 22
- detection rate *107*
- patient 37
  - pathway of care of 37
- spreads 29
- tests, type of 50
- traditional management of 29

Candida infections 151
Cantlie's line 87, 88
Capsule endoscopy 85
Carbohydrate 149
- drinks 125

Carcinoembryonic antigen 68, 117
- role of 118

Carcinoid syndrome 84, 85
Carcinoid tumours 84
Carcinoma 139
Cardiac failure 173
Cardiopulmonary exercise test 206
Cardiovascular insufficiency 37
Care, perioperative 171
Caregiver strain 78
CAR-T cell therapy 32
Catecholamines, enhances actions of 128
Catheterisation 165
CDH1 mutations 63
Cell
- cycle 19, 21, *21*
- death 21
- division 19
- multiplying 25
- number of malignant looking 26
- of Cajal 83
- replicate 21
- theory, third principle of 20
- therapy 33

Central adiposity 64
Central catheter lines, peripherally inserted 150

Central lines, complications of 151
Central venous catheter 150
Cerebral blood flow, autoregulation of 182
Chemical pneumonitis 148
Chemoprevention 65
Chemoradiotherapy, postoperative 72
Chemotherapeutic agents, classification of 32
Chemotherapy 29, 31, 38, 75, 76, 116
 adjuvant 76, 96
 complications 78
 perioperative 71
 postoperative 72
 role of 114
Child–Pugh score 92
Chi-square test 3
Cholangiocarcinoma 92
Chromogranin A 85
Cimetidine 206
Clark's staging *162*
Claude Couinaud classification 87
Clinical guidelines 16
Clodronate 59
Cohort study, prospective 8
Colloid goitre 129
Colon, anatomy of *98*
Colonic blood supply *112*
Colonic resections *112*, *113*
Colonoscopy 118, 121
Colorectal cancer 102, 107, 125
 complications of 114
 management of 111
 presentation 107
 risk of *100*
 staging of *34*, 109
 survival after *119*
 survival of 119
 TNM staging of *111*
 tumourigenesis, molecular basis of 102
Colorectal disease 98
Colorectal malignancy, presentation of *108*
Columnar epithelium 64
Combining lignocaine 176
Compound naevi 162
Computed tomography colonogram 107
Conformal radiotherapy 31
Confusion 179
Constitutional symptoms 66
Conventional endoscopy 85
Core biopsy 48
Corticosteroids 32
Corticotropin-releasing hormone 156
Critical appraisal 9, 16
Crohn's colitis 84
Crohn's disease 144
Cross-sectional study 8
Curling's ulcer 165
Cushing reflex 182
Cuthbertson response 152
Cyclo-oxygenase 175

D

D1 dissection 80
D1 resection 80
D2 dissection 80
D2 resection 80
Data and analysis 3
De novo mutation 27
Dead space air ventilation 173
Death
 causes of 37
 with cancer, causes of 36
Decarboxylation 131
Deep vein thrombosis 14
Dendritic cell 28
Depression 78
Dermal lumps 158
Dermal naevi 161
Diamond 12
 locations of *12*
Diclofenac sodium 175
Dietary factors 64
Digital rectal examination 109, 121
Disappearing liver metastases 117
Distorted architecture 46
Double balloon endoscopy 85
Duct
 carcinoma 43
  in situ 43, 58
 papilloma 42
Dukes' staging 110
Duodenal cancer 66

Duodenum 62
Dysphagia 66, 67, 77
Dysplasia 64, 65, 104
  classification of 65
  high-grade 104
  low-grade 104
Dyspnoea 171, 179

E

Early-stage invasive breast cancer 51
Ebb phase 152
Ectopic testis 169
Electrosurgery, popularisation of 205
Embryology 168
Emerging risk factors 64
Endocrine
  orchestra, control of *155*
  response 152
    pathway *156*
Endoscopic diagnosis 65
Endoscopic mucosal resection 65
Endoscopic retrograde cholangiopancreatography 92, 94
Endoscopic stenting 72
Endoscopic stents 77
Endoscopic techniques 70
Endoscopic therapy 65
Endoscopic ultrasound 71, 92, 95
  examination 92
Endoscopy 94
  screening beyond 73
Enhanced recovery after surgery 125
Enteral feeding, complications of 148
Enteral nutrition 147
  delivery of 148
Environmental factors 63
Epidermal growth factor receptor 32
Epidural anaesthesia 177, 178
Epidural analgesia 177
Epidural infusion 177
Epigastric mass 66, 67
Estrogen receptor 36
Evidence-based practice 16, *16*
Exfoliative cytology 26
Exocrine pancreatic tumours *94*
Exomphalos
  major 170
  minor 170
Experiential case-based learning 180
External beam radiation therapy 76
Extracolonic manifestations 101
Extracorporeal membrane oxygenation 179

F

Factors driving cancer 27
Faecal calprotectin 121
Faecal immunochemical test 106, 121
Familial adenomatous polyposis 62, 63
  coli 101
Familial syndromes 73
Fat necrosis 41, 42
Fatty liver, non-alchoholic 89
Fibroadenoma 41
Fibrocystic disease 41, 42
Fine-needle
  aspiration cytology 48, *133*
  biopsy, role of 90
  cytology 30
Fistula formation 77
Flow phase 152, 153
Fluid 165
  accumulation in ileus, reasons for 146
  creep 165
Follicular carcinoma 134, 135, *135*
Forest plot 11
Fortner operation 96
  types 96
Full blood count 68
Functional impairments 75
Funnel plot 13, *13*
Fusobacterium nucleatum 64

G

Gabapentin 175
Gallbladder carcinoma 93
Galleri test 30
Gastrectomy 79, *79*
  subtotal 79
  types *79*
Gastric cancer 62, 63, 66, 72, 73
  management of 71
  survival in 75
  TNM staging for *69*
Gastric contents, aspiration of 148

Gastric dilatation 165
Gastric tumours, laparoscopic assessment for 71
Gastric ulcers 204
Gastrointestinal bleeding 182
Gastrointestinal reflux disease 62
Gastrointestinal stromal tumour 83, 84
Gastrointestinal system 174
Gastrointestinal tract 83, 84
Gastrojejunostomy 205
Gastro-oesophageal cancer 61
    categories of 70
    staging of *35*
Gastro-oesophageal reflux disease 62, 64
    symptoms 64
Gastro-oesophagoscopy 204
Gastroschisis 170
Gastroscopy 73
Gaussian curve 4
Gaussian distribution curve *4*
General paediatric surgery 167
General plastic surgery 158
Genes, role of 102
Genetic factors 132
Genetic mutations 27
Genetic status 50
Genetic syndromes 62, 63
    risk factors of 100
Genetic testing 73
Genome, guardian of 21
Genomic factors 117
Germline mutations 27
Glucagon 153
Gluconeogenesis 144, 145
Glycogenolysis 145
G-proteins 174
Grave's disease 129, 131
Gubernaculum 168
Gylcogenolysis 144
Gynaecomastia 41, 42

H

Haematemesis 66
Haemicolectomy, right 111
Haemorrhage 77, 134
Haemorrhagic phenomena 37
Haggitt levels *106*
Hartmann's operation 114
Hartmann's procedure 113, 183
Hashimoto's disease 129
Hayflick limit 22
HELA cells 22
Helicobacter pylori 61, 73
    infection 28, 63
Hemi-thyroidectomy 133
Hepatectomy, partial 91
Hepatic complications 151
Hepatic resection 116
Hepatic vein
    middle 88
    right 88
Hepatitis
    B 89
    C infection 89
Hepatobiliary malignancies 87
Hepatocellular carcinoma 89, 92
HER2 29, 32, 36, 46, 50
    targeted therapy 76
Herceptin 32
Hereditary non-polyposis colorectal cancer see also Lynch syndrome 100
Hernia 168
High concentration oxygen therapy 178
High-intensity focussed ultrasound 54
Histamine 174
Histopathology diagnosis 69
Histophysiology 127
Histotripsy 31, 91
Hoarseness 66, 134
Hormonal receptor status 47
Hormone 24
    receptor status 49
    therapy 29, 32
Human epidermal growth factor receptor 2 47
Hungry bone syndrome 141
Hydrocoeles 169
Hydroxy indole acetic acid 84
Hydroxylation 138
Hypercoagulability 67
Hyperglycaemia 157
Hyperparathyroidism 139
    primary 139
    secondary 139, 141
    tertiary 139
Hyperplasia 20, 104, 139

Hypertension 171
Hyperthermic intraperitoneal chemotherapy 78, 117
Hyperthyroidism 131, 139
Hypertrophy 20
Hypotension 179
Hypothalamo-hypophysial axis 155
Hypothesis, alternative 2
Hypoxia 179

I

Ibandronate 59
Ibuprofen 175
Imaging techniques and laparoscopy 71
Immune
  checkpoint inhibitors 33
  system 28
Immuno therapy 32
Immunological response 154
Immunotherapy 117
  surgery 29
In situ neoplasia 43
Infection 24, 37
  prevention of 166
Inflammation 28
Inflammatory breast cancer 44
Inflammatory prostaglandin 175
Infusate 178
Inhibiting sodium channels 176
Inorganic iodine 127
  absorption of 127
Insulin resistance 156, 157
  reduction in 157
Interdisciplinary collaboration 17
Internal beam radiotherapy 31
Interventional surgery 30
Intestinal epithelium 175
Intestinal immune system 146
Intestinal mucosa, primacy of integrity of 145
Intestine thrives 145
Intracranial haemorrhage 181
Intracranial tension, increasing 181
Intraductal papillary mucinous neoplasms 95
Intraoperative ultrasound 117
  role of 117
Invasive carcinoma 43
Iodine deficiency 128
Iron deficiency anaemia 67
Ischaemic bowel fibrillation 185
Ivor Lewis oesophagectomy 82

J

Jaundice 77, 89, 97, 115
Jugulodigastric node 160
Junctional naevi 162

K

Kaplan–Meier curve *13*, 14, 124
Kausch–Whipple pancreatoduodenectomy 96
Ketone bodies 145
Kikuchi levels 106
Klatskin tumour 92
Knudson's two-hit hypothesis 23
KRAS mutation 103

L

Laparoscopic hepatectomy 207
Laparoscopic surgery 72
Large bowel *145*
  gross anatomy of 98
Lead time bias 53, *53*
Left haemicolectomy 111
Left hepatic vein 88
Left supraclavicular node 160
Length of stay 171
Lentigo maligna melanoma 163
Lidocaine 176
Lifestyle risk factors 63
Lipoma 159
  locations of 159
Lipomata 159
Liquid biopsy 74
  tests 30
Liver
  anatomy of 87
  function tests 68
  functional anatomy of *88*
  malignant tumour of 88
  metastases 77, 115
  schematic functional anatomy of *88*
  transplant 92
  transplantation 91

Lobular carcinoma 43
  in situ 43, 44
Local anaesthetic drugs 176
Local complications 77
Localised disease 74
Locoregional disease 54
Locoregional therapies 116
Low-concentration oxygen 178
Lucid interval 181
Luminal A 48
Luminal B 48
Luminal classification, prognostic impact of 48
Lumps 46
Lung metastases 117
Lymph node 160
  dissection 133
Lymphomas 62, 84, 86
Lympho-vascular invasion 48
Lynch syndrome 62, 63

M

Macronutrient 149
Malnutrition 78, 144
  universal screening tool 142
MALT lymphoma 62
Mammography 46
Management strategies 65
Mann–Whitney U test 3
Margin of error 4, 6, *7*
Marginal artery of Drummond 99
Marjolin's ulcer 163
Masses 46
Maternal oestrogen 43
Meckel's diverticulum 182, *183*
Meckel's scan 182
Medical evidence, levels of 14
Medullary carcinoma 44, 135
Medullary thyroid cancer *136*
Melaena 66
Melanoma 119, 162
  superficial spreading 163
  types of 163
Memory loss 179
Mesenteric artery
  inferior 98
  superior 98
Messenger ribonucleic acid 154
Meta analysis 9, 10, *10*, *11*
Metabolic complications 151
Metabolic rate, regulation of 128
Metabolic response 153
  to injury *153*
  to trauma 152
Metabolic syndrome 64
Metabolism, impact on 144
Metastasis 81
  management of 115
Metastatic complications 77, 115
Metastatic work 46
Methotrexate 31, 32, 38
Microbiome 146
  alterations 64
Microcalcifications 46
Micronutrients 150
Microsatellite instability 22
Milan criteria 92
Minimally invasive surgery 72
Mismatch repair genes 21
Mitotic inhibitors 32
Modern abdominal surgery 80
Mohs surgery 163
Monoclonal antibody 76
  therapy 32
Monro–Kellie doctrine 181
Morbidity 172
Morphological anatomy 87, *87*
Mortality 172
Mucinous carcinoma 44
Mucinous cyst neoplasms 95
Mucosal layer 110
Multidisciplinary teams 36
Multiglandular hyperplasia 141
Multinodular goitre 129, 130
Multiorgan failure 185
Multiple endocrine neoplasia 139
Multiple neurofibromatosis 160
Mutations 28
  functional consequences of 28
  gain of function 28
  loss of function 28

N

Naevus 161
Naso-gastric feeding 147
National Confidential Enquiry into Patient Outcome and Death 171

National Surgical Adjuvant Breast and Bowel Project 57
Nausea 66
Neoadjuvant chemotherapy 76
Neoadjuvant therapy 55
Neoplasia 20, 22
Neoplastic lesions, types of 43
Nerve fibres transmit pain, types of 174
Neural sheath tumours, benign 159
Neuroendocrine tumours 84, 86
Neurofibroma 159
- types of *160*

Neurofibromatosis 160
Neurologically mediated sympathetic response 152
NEWS score 173
Nipple discharge 41
Nodes *61*, 81
Nodular melanoma 163
Non-alcoholic steatohepatitis See also metabolic dysfunction associated steatotic liver disease 89
Non-invasive screening, expansion of 74
Nonsteroidal anti-inflammatory drugs 175
Non-urgent referral 67
Normal squamous epithelium, replacement of 64
Nottingham prognostic index 49
Nucleus, size of 26
Null hypothesis 2, 3, 6
Number needed to treat 14
Nutrients, absorption of *145*
Nutritional complications 78
Nutritional requirement 149
Nutritional status 71
Nutritional support 72
- assessment and need of 142
- types of 147

O

Obesity 61, 64
Observational studies 8
Obstructive symptoms 66
Odynophagia 66
Oesophageal adenocarcinoma, progression to 65
Oesophageal cancer 62, 66, 72, 81, *82*
- TNM staging for *69*

Oesophagectomy 65, 81
- three-field 82

Oesophagitis 78
Oesophagogastric cancer *70*
Oesophagogastroduodenoscopy 70, 73
Oesophagus 62
Oestrogen receptor 47
Olovnikov theory 22
Omnis cellula et cellula 20
Oncogenes 28, 102
Oncology 19
Opiate 174
- free infusion 177

Organ invasion 37
Organic iodine 127
- with tyrosine, combination of 127

Oxygen 178
- therapy 178

P

P53 19, 21
- gene 102

Paget's disease 44
- breast 35

Pain
- abdominal 107
- control, postoperative 173
- management 72
- physiology of 173
- reduces 174

Palliation 97
Palliative care, role of 75
Palliative chemotherapy 76
Palliative radiotherapy 78
Palpation 161
Pancreas 61
- anatomy of *93*
- gross anatomy of 93

Pancreatic cancer 93, 97, **97**
- survival rates in 97

Pancreatic cysts 95
Pancreatic malignancies 93
Pancreaticoduodenectomy 86
Papanicolaou smear 27, 30
Papillary carcinoma 44, **135**, 184
- thyroid 132

Paracetamol 174
Paracolic gutters 99

Parafollicular cells 131
Parametric data 3
Paraneoplastic syndromes 67
Paraphimosis 168
Parathormone 137, **139**
    actions of 137
Parathyroid
    adenoma 202
    disease 137
    glands 141
    injury 134
Parenteral nutrition 150
    access for 150
Paris classification *104*
Parkland formula 165
Pemberton's sign 130
Percutaneous endoscopic gastrostomy 78
    tubes, complications of 149
Percutaneous transhepatic cholangiogram 93
Performance score 71
Peritoneal carcinomatosis 117
Peritoneum 98
Persistent dyspepsia 67
Peutz–Jegers syndrome 62, 63
Pharmacological therapy 65
Phimosis 167
Phyllodes tumours 41, 42, 44
Physiological stress 129
Physiology 144, 152
Physiotherapy 173
Plasma *138*
Platelet aggregation
    function 175
    reducing 175
Pneumonia 173
Polyp 103, *104*
    depressed **106**
    malignant 106
    pedunculated **106**
Polyp-cancer
    epithelial sequence 104
    progression *103*
    sequence 103, *105*
Portal vein 88
Positron emission tomography 46, 69
    computed tomography 71, 95
Posthitis 168
Prague classification system 65
Predict breast tool *57*
Prilocaine hydrochloride 176
PRISMA 10
Processus vaginalis testis 169
Proctoscopy 121
Progesterone receptor 36
    positive 47
Protein 149
Proton beam therapy 31
Proton-pump inhibitors 2, 206
Pseudoaneurysm 180
Psychological complications 78
Psychosocial impact 75
Pulmonary metastases 78
P-value 5
    large 6
    small 6
Pylorus preserving technique 95
Pyrexia 174

Q

Quality of life 147

R

Radiation pneumonitis 78
Radical' surgery 31
Radioactive iodine therapy 134
Radioembolisation 116
Radiofrequency ablation 65, 91
Radioisotope scanning 132
Radiotherapy 29, 31, 38, 75
    complications 78
    role of 114
    types of 31
Randomised controlled trials, meta-analysis of 11
RAS mutations 102
Receptor status 46
Rectal artery, superior 98
Rectal bleeding 120
    management of 120
Rectal cancers 113
    laparoscopic resection of *122*
Rectus sheath catheter 178
Recurrent laryngeal nerve 130, 134

Refeeding syndrome 149
Reflux
  disease 63
  symptoms 67
Regional variation 62
Relative risk reduction 15
Renal function 175
Resection *112*
  extended 96
  margin 80
Respiratory failure 37
Respiratory system 174
Retractile testis 169
Retrospective cohort study 8
Retrosternal pain 66
Risk-benefit analysis 16
Robotic assisted surgery 72
Robotic hepatectomy 207
Robotic surgery 207, **207**
Rod-lens
  endoscopes 206
  system 206
Rule of nine **164**, 165

S

Sarcoma 42, 86
Schistosoma mansoni 89
Schwannomatosis 160
Scientific method, principal steps of 7
Sclerosing cholangitis, primary 92
Sebaceous cysts 158
Secreted fluids 146
SEER survival **119**
Selective internal radiotherapy 116
Sentinel node 51
  biopsy 51, 55
Sepsis 173, 185
Serous cystadenoma 95
Serum
  calcium level 137, 140
  carcinoembryonic antigen levels 118
Sessile polyps **106**
Sestamibi scan 140
Shallow breathing 173
Shield test 30
Shrapnel injury 180
Sigmoid colectomy 111
Sigmoidoscopy 121
Single germline mutation 102
Skin
  lumps 158
  melanoma of 162
Small bowel **145**
  cancer **83**
  malignancies 83
Small intestine 83
  malignancy, types of **84**
Smoking 24, 63
Social complications 78
Solitary adenoma, management 130
Solitary goitre 129
Solitary nodule 129
Somatic mutations 27
Spontaneous mutation 22
Squamous cell
  cancer, chemoradiotherapy for 120
  carcinoma 62, 163
Staging systems 69
Standard deviation 4, *4*
Standard infusion 177
Staphylococcus 166
Stereotactic ablative radiotherapy 91
Stereotactic body radiation therapy 116
Stereotactic radiotherapy 31
Stomach 62
  lies 61
Stress
  fundamental response to 156
  ulcers, prevention of 165
Subareolar lumps 41, 42
Subcutaneous lumps 158
  inspection and palpation of 161
Submucosal penetration **106**
Subungual melanoma 163
Suicide 21
Surgery 29, 95, 133
  complications of 118
  volume of 80
Surgical biopsy 30
Surgical bypass 77
Surgical gastrostomy, complications of 149
Surgical management 111
  early evolution of 30
Surgical outcome risk 172

Surgical patient, nutrition of 142, 144
Surgical treatment 140
Surveillance 97
Symptom overlap 74
Systematic review 8, 10
 of research 16
Systemic inflammatory response 184
Systemic therapy 92

T

Tachycardia 179
 tires 173
Tachypnoea 179
Taenia coli 99
Tamoxifen 58
Targeted therapies 76, 116
Telomeres 22
Testis, descent of 168, *169*
Therapy
 complications of 78
 modes of 29
 type of 55
Thromboembolic deterrent 14
Thromboembolic phenomena 37
Thyroglobulin, storehouse of 127
Thyroglossal cyst 184
Thyroid
 cancers of 131, 132, 134, 136
 disease 126
 function 129
  tests 129
 gland
  anatomy of *126*
  lateral aberrant 132
 lobectomy 130
 ultrasound, role of **133**
Thyroidectomy
 completion of 133
 partial 133
 subtotal 130, 131
Thyroid-stimulating hormone 127, 156
Thyrotropin-releasing hormone 127, 156
Thyroxine 127
 doses of 135
 production of 127
 release 127
 T4, actions of 128
TNM
 category **95**
 staging 81, **133**
 system 34
Tobacco and alcohol use 64
Topoisomerase inhibitors 32
Torsion testis 184
Total body surface area **164**
Total gastrectomies 79
Total mesorectal excision 122, 125
Total parenteral nutrition 78, 150
Total thyroidectomy 130, 133
Transabdominal plane block 178
Transarterial chemoembolisation 77
Transhiatal oesophagectomy 82
Transversus abdominis plane block 178
Trastuzumab 32
Trauma 152
Triple assessment (breast)
Trousseau's syndrome 67
Tube, malposition of 149
Tubular carcinoma 44
Tumour 81
 biology 74
 grading 26
 growth curve 24
  doubling dormancy *25*
 growth over time *26*
 markers 94
 stage 25, 74
 suppressor genes 28
Two-hit hypothesis *23*
Tyrosine kinase inhibitors 92

U

Ulcer at tip *183*
Ulcerative colitis 84
Umbilicus hernia 170
Undescended testis 168
Upper abdominal pain 67
Upper gastrointestinal
 cancers 76
 tract, anatomy of 60, *60*
Upper gastrointestinal malignancy 60, 63, 66, 72, 74
 complications of 76
 diagnosis and staging of 68

targeted therapy for 75
types of 62
Urinary 5-HIAA
Urinary infection 168
Urinary tract infection 168

V

Vagotomy 204
Vascular endothelial growth factor inhibitors 76
Vena cava, inferior 87, *87*
Vibrissae, singeing of 165
Video camera, invention of 206
Virchow's node 160
Virus 24
Voice fatigue 130
Vomiting 66
von Recklinghausen's disease 160

W

Weight loss 66
unintentional 66
Whipple's operation 96
Whipple's procedure 86
Wilson's disease 89

Z

Zoledronic acid 59
Z-test 3